PHONE IN THE FRIDGE
Five Years with Multiple Sclerosis

BY

LORNA J. MOORHEAD

Pathfinder Publishing, Inc.
120 South Houghton Road
Tucson, Arizona, 85648

PHONE IN THE FRIDGE
Five Years with Multiple Sclerosis

Published By:
Pathfinder Publishing Inc.
120 South Houghton Road
Tucson, Arizona 88748

First printing 2006

Library of Congress Cataloging-in-Publication Data
Moorhead, Lorna J.
        Phone in the Fridge
        p.cm
        Includes bibliographical references
ISBN 978-0934793-75-9
Price $14.95
1. Medical - Psychological Aspects

PHONE IN THE

Five Years with Multiple Sclerosis

BY

LORNA J. MOORHEAD

CONTENTS

Acknowledgements

To Frances who took the time to point out my mistakes.

To Bill who decided I was worth another shot.

To Judith for all her advice.

To my neurologist and his staff who put up with my questions and antics.

To my family and friends for believing in me.

And most of all to my MS MOMS who remain a source of inspiration, support, and love.

This book is dedicated to Mark.

You changed diapers, cooked dinner,

and kept chaos in check so I could

meet my deadline.

I love you.

~Lorna

The Other Lorna

By Mark, Mr. Lorna, and/or "The Husband"

After proofreading this book, and helping Lorna with the first one, I feel compelled to tell you about MY Lorna, and our five years living with MS. First, let me assure you that I am not as amazing as she makes me out to be. I think I have, maybe, a better understanding of my wife's problem than a lot of caregivers that I've met. Why wouldn't I? You try living with an activist and not learn anything.

Activist. That's a good word for Lorna. If she's not writing a book, she's running a website, or taking on the Power Company. Nothing like that going on? Then she finds some new and exciting way to help others. And wear herself out in the process.

Sure, these last five years have seen some hard times. But I've never been bored. For us, life is always changing. There is always some new challenge to overcome, a new adventure to have, or a new book to write.

Lorna is worth it. We can't always climb hills like we used to, and forget biking. But there are new paths to explore. Maybe we can't climb the hill together, but we can still walk in the park. Watching Lorna try to slither into a sexy black gown can be very comical, but she still tries, and that counts.

Being Lorna's caregiver (By the way, I hate that term.) has only helped me see the truly amazing person she is on the inside. I can compare her to being inside our house on a hot summer day. It's not the outside of the house where the sun beats down and you sit in the heat that makes life comfortable. Instead, it is the inside of the house, on the cozy chair right next to the air-conditioning that makes my life cozy. It is right there, with the person that Lorna is inside...that I know I am comfortable and cozy. I have met a lot of caregivers who feel the same way about their mate. If you find yourself in my shoes someday, stop and look inside the house at all the things in your life that really are important.

Lorna does a lot and I find that I have to remind her to follow her own advice sometimes. Slow down. Rest, and DO put off until tomorrow. But like any good activist, she never seems to follow her own advice. MS has changed Lorna, but she is not defeated in her life. And the disease has far from defeated this family. I attribute this to Lorna, who still works at what's important to us: our children's well-being and our relationship. I will always love her.

Maybe the dishes aren't done. Maybe I have to do a few loads of pink laundry, but Lorna is always there for us. What really counts? That we eat dinner on paper plates? Or is it time together with your mate and your family?

Introduction
5 Years Later

Here's a comment pitched to me in a review of my first book, *Coffee in the Cereal: The First Year with Multiple Sclerosis.* The reviewer insinuated that if you weren't "depressed or angry about your MS," then you should not read my book. I was flabbergasted. The idea that any MSer is entirely at peace, speaking cheerfully about MS was as foreign to me as Britney Spears wearing a shirt that actually covers her navel. Does such a shirt exist? Does such a sufferer exist?

Captivated by this happy reviewer's opening toss, I read on. Chills ran the length of my body. Either that or it was the air-conditioning. In the next breath, the reviewer claimed that she was not defined by MS. "This books acts as if your MS will begin to define who you are." An enlightening, but unhelpful, pitch to be sure. Funny, I did not search out the reviewer to thank them for showing me the error of my ways.

Instead, I laughed. I laughed like I did the day my eldest son Stephan told me that the Easter Bunny laid eggs because the TV told him so. I shook my head in amazement. How many times in my life since my diagnosis have I heard the phrase: "Denial is not a river in Egypt?"

Moving on and not giving much thought to MS, that is easy for sufferers with little or no daily symptoms. People have died, you know, and only in an autopsy did doctors discover a brain riddled with MS lesions. For those with a little fatigue and no other symptoms, life does go on. In their mind, and in the mind of that reviewer, life should go on merrily for others with

MS as well. The disease should not take over, move in, or define our lives.

I'm not saying that, everyday, my MS tears my life apart. In fact in the last five years, I have learned that many of my original views about MS were a bit overblown, as that should be for someone newly diagnosed with a life altering disease. But I am saying that no matter how you slice it, MS has changed my life and who I am, forever. People can claim that they will not let MS define them. Great. Nevertheless, when you have gone from Aerobic Aphrodite to the Countess of the Couch, you have to admit, you've been collected, categorized, and defined. Whether it is the fact that I now take shots most days or that sometimes I can't hop on one foot with my son, MS has changed my life.

After five years with MS, I believe I have moved up (or down depending on perspective) the ladder of MSers from beginning to intermediate. I am in no way as seasoned as people who have had MS for ten years, but I have moved past running about like a chicken with no head. (At least on good days.)

When I was first diagnosed with MS, I reacted strongly. MS moved into my life and took up residence like an annoying relative. During this time, every twitch of a muscle, every ache or pain, became a possible MS complication. I developed a type of MS-hypochondria. Each day my MS defined every waking moment. Each time something odd happened, I knew it was my multiple sclerosis acting up and that my life was ending. Yes, I know how uninformed that was, but that was how drastic it felt.

Five years later, I can look back at this microscopic view of my condition and laugh. Laugh, and question my sanity at the time. In retrospect, I know why I reacted with such intense focus. I was faced with a concept that most people hate to consider: having no control. I lost my choice about how I wanted to live the next 50 years of my life. I had to adapt my definition of the future, and my definition of myself for my MS. I was being defined without a choice, and I hated it. So the best therapy for this, as it has always been throughout my life, was to write.

I sat down and poured out how I felt. Told stories of situations and tried to make some sense and fun out of it. I looked for the proverbial silver lining to what felt like the end of the world to me. I dug my heels in and sassed the people who told me I looked great. I thumbed my nose at unhelpful health professionals and state workers. I took all my anger, confusion, and hopelessness and poured it out on paper. In doing so, I began to find hope, humor, and light. A new definition of my self and my future. A future where I may not have complete control over my body, but I did have control over how I looked at things.

In my mind, not letting my MS define my life now would simply be denial. Denial of who I am. Besides, who would want to ignore blissfully the roller coaster that is MS? When you let MS define you, the definition changes everyday! One day, you're almost back to your old self, lifting weights and walking fast on a treadmill. The next day you're doing the best imitation of a ground sloth. MS may be many bad things, but one thing it is not is DULL. But get over it and act as if it never happened? HA!

Whether I am bemoaning my existence, screaming at God, educating others about the disease, or kicking auto-immune butt at the gym, MS still defines me. It's there in every compensation I have made to live with my body. On good days and bad days, and even days when I don't think about it at all. And by the way, I can say that there are days when MS never enters my mind. But my MS is still there, determining how each day will begin and end.

If you get over it or move on with life as if the multiple sclerosis did not exist, you are puttin' on the blinders. Some lucky people have nary a symptom. Working nine to five and carrying out their lives is no problem. However, even these people along with the rest of us face relapse day, when a new symptoms pops up, when we are hit smack in the face with MS, and the limits of our bodies. If a person has denied the possibility that MS can interfere with life, get ready for a nasty revelation. Relapse Happens.

Is it healthy to spend each waking moment focused on your MS? Maybe not. But I say it is okay for a newly diagnosed person to go right ahead and do it. It is part of the process. Is it any healthier to act like it's no big thing? One of my rants, in MS MINDS, a newsletter I sporadically come out with, I spoke of MS as a beehive in the corner. Don't run around screaming about the bees. Certainly don't bash at the hive with a broom. But be sure you are aware that the hive is there. And be aware of what it can do. Ignoring the beehive will get you stung. Awareness can be difficult, but over time leaves you much better prepared emotionally and physically for that bee sting.

So get over it? No. Get on with it? Yes.

What follows is a series of rants and articles that I have written in the past five years regarding multiple sclerosis. Just like the disease there is no rhyme or reason to their organization. It is a journal, if you will, of different situations I have come across, emotions I have dealt with, and advice I have given to others like myself.

I'm not going to tell you how to become one with your MS. I'm not going to launch into complicated medical explanations of what Multiple Sclerosis is or tell you how to cure it. And I'm definitely not going to regale you with stories of how I conquered the evil dictator of a small third world country all the while taking my shots. What I will do is:

·   Impart a bit of knowledge on living with MS.

· Give odd insight into situations we've all encoun
tered.

· Talk about scandalous subjects such as blad
der control and alternative therapies.

· And most importantly, give you the ability, even if just
for a few moments, to find a horrible diagnosis horribly funny.

CHAPTER I

Lorna's Diagnostic Saga:

A Sonata in 6 Parts

All in My Pretty Little Head

But you don't look sick...

I can remember exactly when the first symptom hit. Not the symptoms that come and go that you brush off thinking, "It was just a fluke." I mean the first symptom that told me something was wrong.

I had been feeling fatigued. But having just dealt with a nasty falling out with a roommate, I figured the fatigue was stress. I had also quit exercising because I was constantly tired. All this I brushed off with the usual explanation of stress or depression.

I was alone in the house because my eldest son, who was two at the time, was with his grandmother, and my husband was away at work. He works weekends at Renaissance Fairs and was usually gone from Friday-Sunday night. I was at the computer on a chat channel during this weekend, wasting away my hours, when I noticed my hands were shaking. My fingers became hard to direct. I began making typos, and then I was vibrating so badly that I couldn't type. I felt confused and weary. People online told me it must be low blood sugar.

Taking their advice, I gobbled down some food and waited for this miracle cure to stop my hands. It didn't. I decided to go to my room and rest. I remember lying on the bed thinking that the soft jolts to the mattress from my hands, and now lower arms, felt like one of those massaging hotel beds. I even relaxed enough to giggle about it. After about an hour or two the tremors slowed to a stop. The next day I called the doctor.

Within a week, we were convinced I was hypoglycemic. I bought a blood sugar testing machine and walked around with sore fingertips from tracking my blood sugar. I changed my diet and was sure that the doctor was right. Wrong. I continued to have problems. Besides the shaking, I became confused, agitated, and forgetful. I was always tired. Nevertheless, since I was 23 and very healthy, it simply had to be blood sugar. Or anxiety.

That was the diagnostic choice of the next doctor we saw. We had just moved back to the city after living rather secluded in the hills above Sacramento. So when I went in with my explanation, she told me that I was anxious and stressed after the move. After having panic attacks at age 18, I was well aware of what I felt like when I was anxious and this WAS NOT it. I bluntly told her so. To appease me she gave me a brief neurological examination. You know. Touch your nose. Flop your hand back and forth in your palm as if mimicking a dying fish. So I flopped my hands, tried to walk on my heels, and attempted to touch my nose with my eyes closed. I almost fell over. To my relief, she now believed it wasn't my nerves. My dismay was simultaneous, because she thought it was something worse. She got me an appointment to see a neurologist. A neurologist? Now, this was scary. What could be so seriously wrong that it would require the once over by a person specializing in the brain? Obviously my diagnosis was no longer hypoglycemia.

I wasn't due to see the neurologist for a month. In that month, I had already planned a trip to London with my mother, all expense paid by my mum of course. I wondered if I was allowed to go. The doctor told me I was in no serious danger. "You are fine to take the trip," she said. No serious danger? Danger of what? This early in the game, I had not learned to ask the doctor for exacting explanations. Seeing as how I was in "no serious danger," I went. At this point, I was beginning to frighten myself with thoughts of a brain tumor, or because of the tremors, epilepsy. I was betting on epilepsy. Yet, seizures or no I was determined to see the Tower of London.

The flight was fine. I didn't get much sleep, but who can in those tiny seats? I was completely exhausted when we arrived. It took awhile before the hotel man came to pick us up and dragged us to our hotel. Once there, we took a short nap and then forced ourselves up to have some dinner. Besides being tired and cranky, everything seemed great. The food was better than expected, I had always heard English food was bland, and I loved spending time with my mother. I was exhausted but thoroughly ready to enjoy two weeks in England. Later that night, after a telephone conversation with my husband, I felt a bit homesick and emotionally distraught. I remember thinking that I felt so tired, so drained that I didn't know if I would ever get my energy back. Deciding I just needed some sleep, I dozed off.

It was exactly one hour later. I opened my eyes and looked around my house. I could not understand why my husband had moved the furniture and I was furious. I looked around the room and tried to find him. I went to the bedroom door and opened it. I did not see our kitchen but instead the long hallway of the hotel. I shut the door and leaned against it trying to clear my head. It was tight as if someone had strapped a vice on it and everything in the room seemed odd, tilted. Becoming overwhelmed with nausea, I lurched into the bathroom.

I don't remember exactly what happened, but I must have lowered myself to the floor, as that is where I remember being next. I had finally realized where I was and I had lost bladder control. Scared, embarrassed, and sobbing, I began to run the bath water in the attempt to calm myself and to hide the evidence of my incontinence from my mother. I prayed she wouldn't wake up, and then I prayed I wouldn't die. I know that sounds silly but I had no clue as to what was going wrong. I felt completely betrayed by my body and my life. It felt as if suddenly a giant force was sucking me under and I was powerless to stop it. I began thinking about my son and my husband at home, and panicked further. I was terrified.

Now in a full-blown panic attack, I lost any hope of hiding everything from my mother and woke her up. It was 3 a.m. I sobbed and told her what had happened. She was very confused and tried to calm me by reassuring me it was just jet lag and that I was over tired. I called my husband and sobbed to him. I told him I wanted to come home. He calmly told me that was impossible and to get some sleep. About dawn, I fell into a fitful sleep.

Within 48 hours, I was back home. Three days later, I was in the emergency room, with another bout of incontinence. I also kept having what I called "waves." It would feel as if I was about to black out. I would not be able to speak through them and the best way I could describe the feeling to doctors was as if my brain was having a brownout. I kept telling people, "I feel like I am going backward, like I am becoming a baby again or becoming mentally handicapped." I had trouble walking, and the rooms always seemed to move around me.

After 13 hours in the emergency room, one CT scan, and another neurological exam, all they could tell me was that my right side was weak and that I didn't have a tumor. Gee, thanks. I was left to wait for the neurologist appointment. Little did I know the worst was yet to come.

I supposed I knew the answer to the question, "Am I Crazy?"

Am I Crazy?

Filled with anticipation about discovering what was going wrong with me, the time for my first neurologist appointment came. I knew that this man could tell me what was wrong with me. Clutching Mark's arm, we made our way into the exam room. When we first entered the office, I was a bit taken aback when I noticed that I was the only native English speaker in the room besides my husband. Determined not to get my hopes down about the type of care I might receive from a neurologist that did not cater to English speaking clients, I ignored the nagging doubts that were whispering through my head.

The neurologist entered the room and instantly told me to get off the table and sit in a chair by him. He seemed rough. I became nervous. Next, he asked me to tell him what was happening. As I fumbled through my story trying to keep my thoughts from straying, he kept cutting me off and finishing my sentences for me, sometimes incorrectly.

"Why were you slurring?" he asked

"Well I was only slurring that day because I had bit my tongue in my sleep and my tongue was swollen."

"Have you done that before?"
"Yes, but not often, just sometimes I clamp my mouth down so hard and my tongue gets in the way. I have never seriously hurt myself. I think I do it out of stress. Besides that is not why I am here." I noticed him scribbling on his paper and saw the words: "History of tongue biting."

Next, he cut off my story about my trip to London with my mother, and told me to get on the exam table. By this point, I was horribly nervous and felt that this man did not believe me. He seemed so cold and distant. I did not believe for a second that he had even heard what I said.

The examination was exactly like the one they had given me in the emergency room. Except this neurologist made me do everything faster and with my eyes closed. It reminded me of that joke about how Ginger Rogers did everything Fred Astaire did except backwards and in high heels. My limbs continued to tremor and every task he asked me to perform seemed very difficult. I remembered how graceful I had once been in dance class, and felt miserable.

When he was done, he briskly told me to put on my shoes and then revealed to me, as if some spiritual being had just whispered it in his ear, that I had epilepsy. The neurologist scheduled an EEG and sent me on my way, letting me know the DMV would take away my license temporarily until they discovered if I was truly having seizures. I didn't get my driver's license back until three years later, 2002.
Mark and I went home shocked. Epilepsy. There had been some discussion, after we ruled out hypoglycemia and a tumor, of neurological Lyme disease, since I had been diagnosed with Lyme at 15, and then most likely cured. Epilepsy had entered my mind, but I had still thought that to have epilepsy I must have these seizures, none of which I had experienced. I felt certain that the neurologist had focused his whole probable diagnosis on one fact, my swollen tongue, and nothing else I had told him.

In my wait for the EEG, I began to research Epilepsy on the Internet. My family was confused. I was still fatigued every single day. My nerves were at the breaking point. Off and on since the fated night in London, I had begun to experience what I called "waves."

In these system brown-outs, everything around me would fade momentarily and then come back in. I would never loose consciousness, or sight, but I would barely be able to talk through these spells and felt as if I might pass out. To this day, I do not feel as if I am explaining this correctly. I just wish sometimes my friends and family could experience one of these waves. At home, I was dropping things, slurring, forgetting bill payments, and having uncontrollable mood swings.

On the day of the EEG, I was concerned that if I did have epilepsy, it would not show up. I had been reading everything I could on the Internet and had found more than once that women who were having PMS tended to have their epilepsy act up, whereas women who were menstruating seemed to have fewer episodes or none. I was on my period and was sure that it would mess up the test if I were an epileptic. When the test only lasted a half hour and did not include me falling into a restful sleep (with the construction crew banging away on that particular section of the hospital), I was sure that the results would be negative.

I was right.

Within a few weeks, I was back at the first neurologist's office waiting to hear what he planned to do next. He escorted my husband and me into the room where I promptly handed him some scribbled journal entries I had made in order to try to explain what was happening to me. He took a few seconds to look over the scribbled, messy pages, and then looked at me. I was not as surprised as I thought I might be when the neurologist looked at me coldly, almost cruelly.

"Your EEG came back normal." The look on his face reminded me of a parent confronting a child who has been lying.

"Yes?" I asked quietly, suddenly fearing this man and hating myself for feeling victimized by him.

Chapter 1

"I am thinking that you have lots of stress in your life. I am going to refer you back to your primary care and tell them that you need to see psychiatrist for evaluation," he said coldly.

"What?" I gripped the sides of the chair and thought I would loose consciousness this time. My husband's face turned red. I barely hung on to the small thought that if I yelled at him it would confirm his diagnosis that I was psycho. I tried to slowly get my words out, to rationalize with him. "I admit I have had panic attacks before in my life doctor, but these are not them. The only thing I am anxious about is what is wrong with me."

"Well some people think they are happy. They are wealthy and have good families, yet they still jump off bridges." Jump off bridges? My mouth fell open. He stood up and pushed my journal entries back towards me. "You will want to show these to a psychiatrist," he said pointedly looking at the pages and then removing his hands from them as if they were contaminated. With this, he left.

My diagnosis now? Not epilepsy, but just plain crazy, and I had lost my freedom

Wasn't Spinal Tap a Band?

It was time to find a new neurologist and a second opinion. I retraced my steps back to my primary care and told her she had to find someone else. She listened and displayed some concern over my treatment, but still remained looking at me with guarded eyes as if she was beginning to worry for my sanity. Within the space of a few days, they had given me an appointment with a new neurologist. The quickness with which I got the appointment was astounding. I wondered if someone had been listening all those dark nights that I lay whispering in my mind to anyone who would listen.

The night before seemed to stretch. I lay awake experiencing what I had nicknamed "waves," little brain power surges. One moment I was working fine and then the next everything seemed to slow and loose power, then just when I thought I was going to loose consciousness, everything would come back and I was fine. I would glance at my husband and wonder how tired he was. How convinced was he that I was insane? I felt entirely alone in myself and yet at the same time, I felt even I didn't belong in this body. THIS body was someone else's. Who was controlling my body? I sure had no control. I never knew when I would loose bladder control again, when my hands would start shaking, when my balance would tip, and when my vision would go weird. Grocery store aisles were long halls of brightly colored noise jumping out at me. I would stare at the floor in order to walk straight and not crash. Noise bothered me. I looked and sounded drunk. I began to hate my body. I began to loose faith. Where were my guardian angels? My spirit ancestors? My God? I talked to every deity I could think of, and they all told me to leave a message.

Chapter 1

Mark and I went hand in hand the next morning to face the new neurologist. The blonde smiling man who ushered us back into his office was not what I expected. He listened to my heart with a stethoscope and then plopped behind his desk. I wondered what the heart thing was for, but forced myself to focus on talking and making my point. It seemed I only had a few words out before he started asking quick questions and writing. My mind whirled and feeling as if I was under sedation I tried to reach through the fog and answer him correctly. When he found out that the previous neurologist had only run one test, he became angry.

"What about a spinal tap? Did he do that?" he grumbled.

"N-no. He did just the EEG and told me I was in need of a shrink," I responded, my lips feeling fat. My hands began twitching worse with nervousness added on top of my condition.

"Okay, well we need a spinal tap and an MRI. We will also take some blood tests. You had Lyme disease once?"

"Yes, when I was 15. I understand that Lyme can, in later stages become Neurological Lyme, affecting the brain."

"Well I don't think it's that, but we'll run a Lyme titer and check." With that, he hopped up and escorted us to the front desk to set up the tests.

He was willing to do tests, and he was willing to make a thorough diagnosis! A feeling of relief, of fat cherubs singing above my dizzy head, rushed through me and then...a spinal tap? The idea made me want to crawl back into bed and hide. I went home and had a drink. In the middle of the afternoon, to calm myself down. Up until then, the only time my back had ever been graced by the presence of a needle, was during for the epidural when I had my first son. "Yeah. But this doesn't make you go numb all over and feel great," I thought.

While waiting for the spinal tap, I began to be consoled by everyone about my mystery condition. It didn't help much. Many people told me that it was only stress. Some told me, "I do those silly things too and nothing was wrong with me." I would nod, feel angry, and have another pint of ice cream. I KNEW my body and MY BODY was a traitor. It wasn't stress. It wasn't senility. It wasn't my imagination.

The Hokey Pokey

The morning for my lumbar puncture, or spinal tap, had come. I sat in the hospital in-patient area dressed in a little white gown that was thankfully made of cloth not paper, otherwise it would be falling off while I clutched at it in embarrassment. As it was, I was constantly tucking the edges around me so that I did not flash the nurses. Mark sat next to the hospital bed, reading a magazine with one hand while his other patted my thigh. Determined to be brave, educated from my studies on the Internet regarding the procedure, I listened to my neurologist as he talked to the nurses. Then suddenly burst into tears.

"I can't do it." I gasped and Mark abandoned his reading to jump up and wrap his arms around me tightly. "I want to go home." Unreasonable fear had swallowed me up and all I could think of was the needle and my bare back.

When she re-entered my curtained "bedroom," the nurse was shocked to find me crying as I had been laughing and talking easily only moments before. Smiling softly she handed me the stuffed toy I had brought with me for comfort. Byron, a shaggy dog, had always accompanied me in times of anxiety from boarding school to the birth of my first son. Byron was always propped on my bed or being tackled by my five-year-old son and had come not only represent security, but family. I believed that no one was ever to old to have a comfort item such as a teddy bear or shaggy dog. I tucked the animal under my arm and smiled through my tears. By now, my body was shaking but I felt a reasonable grip on my anxiety. Then the neurologist walked in. I began sobbing again. I felt like a fool and the worst kind of coward. He spared no time with my emotional state, in fact it appeared that this was a common reaction to the idea of having a needle in one's back, so he ordered me to lay down and curl my legs up in the fetal position.

"Let's get this over real quick shall we? There's no reason to be afraid Lorna." His tone was firm, like the one my parents used when I was a child and thought panicking would get me out of a dentist visit. His tone clearly said, "We'll do this with you calm or we'll do this with you freaking out," even if he didn't. Visualizing what I might look like if the hospital staff had to hold me down during the procedure as I screamed and carried on, I relaxed. A little. Mark had been removed from the area and this fact was doing nothing to make me feel better. I'm not sure if the procedure called for it or not but the nurse wrapped an arm over my head and shoulder to keep me still. She leaned her chest down onto me and this bear hug she was giving me helped to keep me calm. It also made it impossible for me to escape. Now that I come to think of it, I'm positive this was standard procedure for spinal taps. I tensed as I felt the cold wipe on my back.

"What a beautiful back you have," my neurologist murmured. Yeah, I bet you say that to all the girls, I thought. For a moment I almost laughed. He continued, "This will be quite fast. Now I am going to use a very tiny needle. First a prick to numb you." I barely felt it, but closed my eyes and began to shake from the adrenaline. "Now there we go, opening pressure is.." I cannot remember the numbers, but envisioned some sort of gauge sticking from a hole in my back like they have on all those pipes in broiler rooms. The thought made me feel like vomiting so I cursed my imagination and clutched Byron.

I opened my eyes and looked up at the wonderful butterfly earrings in the nurse's ears. It is funny what you latch on to and remember in those quick panicked moments of your life. A red shirt, blue and purple butterfly earrings, and the cancer patients who were getting their daily dose of chemo on the other side of the curtains. There was the cheery voice of a woman determined not to let cancer get her down and my guilt for selfishly thinking that I had been the only person in the room suffering.

By now I was getting what I call "woozy" and I told the doctor this. He laughed softly and asked what "woozy" was. As I tried to explain that "woozy" essentially was the nauseous feeling and first sign one gets before passing out, I began to break out in a cold sweat. That was the second sign.

"Are we almost done?" I whispered, shaking and sweating. I was sure if they did not finish soon, I would faint. Funny, that at the time my worst fear was fainting. Fainting might have been an nice alternative to being awake with my imagination taking what was a simple, albeit uncomfortable procedure, and making it a nightmare. The nurse nodded and squeezed me tighter. I could barely feel anything going on behind me, only the touch of the Dr.'s hands every once in awhile and a dull feeling of something poking me in the back. There was no pain. What seemed like 20 minutes could only have been 2, and then it was over.

"There we go. All done. Now roll over on your back and stay that way," my neurologist said, smiling. I noticed some blood on a pad that had been under my back and closed my eyes against another surge of "woozy." My father, who had arrived to be my caretaker for the weekend since Mark would be out of town working, peeked around the curtain. Mark followed him looking sad. I asked for a cold wash-cloth and worried that I might get sick and embarrass myself further. Mark applied the wash-cloth and feeling awful that he had to leave at such a time, kissed me goodbye promising to call as soon as he could. My father was now the one who sat by my bed for the eight hours my neurologist had instructed that I remain flat before going home. It amused both my father and myself that he, who was now 70 (yet fit as a mule) should once again be in charge of nursing me and not vice versa.

At this point I was relieved to be through the worst. In fact the sleepless nights before the procedure and the fear and panic during were the hardest part. I was completely innocent when it came to spinal taps and had no idea what was about to befall me.

Headache My A**!

The nurses sent me home that Friday and told me simply, "If your head hurts lay down." Still feeling woozy and aching from laying on my back all day, my father and I hobbled out of the hospital and headed to his house. We tried to keep me semi-reclined in the car except I kept holding my back arched afraid that touching the seat would send some sort of heinous pain down my spine.

In celebration of my survival, because my father always re-warded making it through rough stuff even if I did cry like a baby and panic, Dad treated me to the best kind of horribly greasy fast food and a movie rental. We then headed to home where I casually reclined, half sitting-half lying on the couch. My head throbbed only once in awhile. By the end of the night I was lying down most of the time. However, I continued to get up and down to raid the fridge for snacks and visit the bath-room.

By Sunday morning, at 5:00 a.m., I could no longer move with-out pain. I'm talking serious pain. I had what I soon learned was a spinal headache. (Headache my a**! It should be re-ferred to as the "my-brain-is-pounding-against-the-inside-of-my-skull-I'm-going-to-vomit-my-ears-are-exploding-my-eyes-hanging-out-of-their-sockets-headache.")

No longer able to sit up, my father called for an ambulance and off we went, back to the hospital. According to the EMT in the ambulance with me, not only was I in pain but instead of my blood pressure sky-rocketing as it should do in pain, mine was dropping. Not a good sign. The hospital staff got me into a bed in the emergency room and told me they were going to start an IV. Why is it they always tell you about something like this and then leave the room for about 10 minutes? I think they sit back somewhere and giggle as your pulse shoots in antici- pation of having a needle rammed into the back of your hand. And I do mean RAMMED. They always send some nurse who must have trained shooting Army men lined in a row. I can picture her waddling down the curtained row in the hospital shoving IV's in and yelling, "Next!"

Soon after my second poke in one weekend, they wheeled me to my own private room upstairs. It was apparent I was going to stay. Soon, my neurologist arrived looking irritated.

"Well I see someone didn't stay down for 24 hours," he growled. My eyes widened.

"No one said to stay down! They said go home and lay down if your head hurts." I became ready to strangle the nurses. He grumbled something about those nurses and then leaned over my head, pulling away my pillow.
"You need to be completely flat. Tomorrow you can go home." With this, he rushed out of the room, hopefully to go behead a nurse.

My father made himself comfortable on the couch and I lay unmoving, my back and head pounding out what might have been Morse code for "You should of stayed down. You should of stayed down." I winced and took advantage of the one vice you can indulge in at hospitals. Drugs.

While loading my IV, the nurse told me that she was giving me only a small amount of the painkiller as it had a "tendency to make people queasy." An hour later a little queasy had me doing my best impression of the Exorcist. Laying sideways on the bed, a metal bowl shoved up to face, my head no longer pounded but was on fire. Next they gave me a little something to handle the nausea. This seemed to have the effect on my thoughts of about six espressos. So while I could not hold open my eyes because the room swam, my brain was racing with thoughts. Too drugged to make sense of things, I panicked. With the panic came the fight or flight syndrome. I became convinced that I had to get away from this horrible hospital. Not feeling any pain, I sat up and begged my father to ask them to "let me go." He asked, only to settle me, and of course they were not going to let me leave. Not able to think clearly and only aware that my mind was racing while my body was numb, I threatened to rip out my IV and walk home. The nurse did not believe me. Plus, she had a look on her face that told me if I did try, she would drag me back by my scruff.

Realizing that just possibly I was not coping well with the effects of the two medications, she talked me through some meditations to calm me and we all waited for the medication to wear off. By nightfall, the insane feeling had begun to lessen and the aches came back full force. My legs and back cramped as if I had spent the day hiking; and the idea of staying the night terrified me. My one consolation was my husband. He was coming back that night. I only worried that he would find our house empty and not know what had happened.

After hearing from his parents that I had been sent to the hospital, he rushed over, still in his renaissance fair clothing, to be by my side and relieve my worn out father. After battling with his possessed daughter, my Dad was quite ready to go home. Calmed by my husband's presence and with the help of a regular old-fashioned sleeping pill, and the Tony Awards on TV, I made it through the night.

The next morning, though my head still ached when I raised it, I was determined to go home. The nurses let me slowly inch my bed to a sitting position and I waited anxiously for my neurologist to come see me. He rushed in as if it had only been ten minutes since he last saw me and not a hideous 24 hours.

He stopped and frowned when he saw me propped up.

"What are you doing up?" he growled.

"The nurses said I could. It's been 24 hours." I felt like I was a child that no-one would believe. My voice even cracked. I clutched my fists in the sheets incensed that I was being blamed for someone else's mistake. He sighed and nodded. I began to wonder if he knew something about this hospital's rate of care that I did not.

"Are you feeling better?" he asked with genuine concern. Now this was a loaded question for me. I felt better compared to my drug ridden nightmare but nowhere near recovered.

"I'm fine," I replied quickly. He arched an eyebrow, I think he knew I just wanted out of there, and then smiled.

"Okay but you go home and STAY down." He wagged a finger at me. I nodded. With that, the wheelchair came in and my exit began. Although I almost fainted from the throbbing which remained, I had now become a bit paranoid of this hospital and wanted OUT. This had not been the touching experience of my first son's birth. This had been Hell. I went home, rested, acknowledged the fact that I now knew more about bed pans than I ever wanted to know, and was comforted by the notion that I would never have to go through that horrible procedure again.

Boy was I in for a shock....

They LOST it?!

"Well the first part of your spinal tap results came back and there were some raised numbers, but the other part which looks for the oligoclonal bands has not come in. It appears the lab has lost the spinal fluid."

For a moment I was not sure I had heard my neurologist correctly. I had been digesting the shock from the fact that "raised numbers" did not sound good and wondering what type of music the Oligoclonal bands play. It was then that I realized these bands seemed very important to my neurologist and that due to the incompetence of the lab, I was most likely going to have another spinal tap. I actually giggled. The helplessness of the situation overwhelmed me and there was nothing to do but find it somehow humorous. I pictured the lab technicians tripping over themselves and barely catching test tubes in a sort of modern day Three Stooges fashion. This image, however angering, was humorous. The world is an unpredictable place. Sometimes I wish it was unpredictable all over someone else.

"That means I have to do it again, doesn't it?" I asked as calmly as I could. I shot a look to my partner who was about to jump off the couch in anger.

"Yes, I would like that. This same lab has done this before and I am going to quit using them. However, I would like that test to be done on the spinal fluid before I make a diagnosis," he said.

Why were these bands so important to him? Well, according to my research on the web, despite the advancements in technology and medical science, it is still very difficult to accurately diagnose Multiple Sclerosis. The symptoms are so wide and varied that the disease can look like many different conditions. The three main tests a neurologist uses to diagnosis MS is an MRI, evoked potential, and a spinal tap.

After a spinal tap, the doctors look for an increase in lymphocytes (a type of white cell), immunoglobins, and the oligoclonal bands. The bands are found by running a test on the spinal fluid called 0 electrophoresis. Abnormal blips, or bands, in the spinal fluid protein are revealed in 80% of the people with Multiple Sclerosis. Therefore, you can see why my neurologist really wanted this test done correctly.

Since my first spinal tap ended with me in the hospital, I was not as eager as he to go hunting for oligoclonal bands. I squirmed in my seat and then asked what he thought my diagnosis might be from the results he did get. He looked back down at the chart and said, "These numbers show signs that something is definitely going on. I am thinking it is possibly Multiple Sclerosis, but there are other diagnoses I want to rule out." I nodded, sighed, and told him to reschedule the test.

"The next test I would like to have done while we are waiting for the authorization for the second puncture is a MRI," he added. I numbly nodded again, the humor of the situation had suddenly left, and the seriousness of my possible diagnosis took its place. He escorted me out of the office and I walked down the hall, numb.

* * * * *

The MRI machine was a tube. It looked to be about 10 feet in length. Although the body of the monster is large and wide, the actual mouth appeared to be about the size of your average cannon opening. Along with its intimidating appearance, came its voice. A consistent humming, that reminded me of the idling engine from that man-eating car in the movie "Christine," based

35

on a book by the master of horror, Stephen King. At this point I was trying not to think of every scary thing he ever wrote, and was asked to lie down and calmly let myself be loaded into its mouth.

After being propelled gently into its belly with a slotted helmet over my face, that not only held my head in place but also had a nifty mirror to let me see my husband at the foot of the machine, I promptly freaked out. Although I must admit that I did not flail my hands or scream, I repeatedly asked for the technician to "pull me out NOW." I had only been inside the machine for about 20 seconds. The test had not even begun. The tongue spit me back out and I sat up, reaching for my husband. This was about the point when I realized that although I had lived for 24 years without knowing it, I was claustrophobic.

With great irritation the technician joined me and my husband in the room and flatly stated that he would give me a few seconds to calm down. My skin was already clammy and the cold chills that ran over my body signaled the beginning of a panic attack. Within moments my ears were ringing and I was hanging my head between my legs to keep from fainting. My husband kept saying something about relaxing and how I needed the test done, while the technician informed me rather curtly, that he would be putting me "back in now." I only shook my head and thought that although newborns seem desperate to crawl back into their mother's womb, I had lost that instinct and had no intention of being "put back in."

Although he acted like it was a vital piece of top-secret government data that was being pried from him in torture, the technician grudgingly informed me that there was the choice of rescheduling the test with Valium. Valium, the little blue (or yellow depending on dosage) pill and my old friend. Valium was the reason I made it home from London after my first spell in one piece. Valium introduced me to my first experience with actually SLEEPING on an airplane. Valium was good. Valium was nice. I understood why people got addicted to Valium. You could have someone inform you of your lover's death while on Valium and you would only smile and say, "Gee. That's too bad."

I rescheduled the test, now marked as "one of those claustro-phobic, anxious wrecks, that needs to be sedated to do a simple test." I asked him if they could put me to sleep with one of those tranquilizer guns you always see on those animal shows, but he did not think it was funny. I went home and informed my family and friends that I had joined the ranks of the "chickens." Yet, somehow it felt more in the ranks of trembling egg yolk.)

The MRI, or Magnetic Resonance Imaging, is not usually a harrowing experience. The MRI machine uses a magnet to take x-ray like pictures of various parts of the body to help with the diagnosis of various medical problems. In the case of Mul-tiple Sclerosis, it is helpful in spotting areas of demyelination, where the protective covering of the nerves has been dam-aged. Most people make it through this test with their confi-dence and self-esteem intact.

When I went the second time, the technician was a woman and very helpful. I figured they reserved her for the nervous patients. When she loaded me into the tube to have my head examined, she showed me that my head was actually close to the opening at the other end. The tube, she pointed out, al-though appearing tiny, was actually large enough to relax my shoulders in, and was equipped with a fan that blew a slight breeze through the machine. Although the MRI examines your head, you will not walk away from the session feeling that your problems have been solved or with a recommendation to read *I'm Okay, You're Okay.*

She offered me a blindfold, which I refused. The next thing I got was some squishy earplugs. You roll them between your fingers and then shove them into your ears. Once inserted, these things bloat, like a lion full of wildebeest, and it is hard to hear anything. I now use them regularly when I need some serious sleep. After placing me into the head cage with the little mirror, she softly asked if I was ready. Thankfully, due to the miracles of Valium, I was.

The test was 30 minutes broken into sections where the machine made weird noises and banging. Mark remained at my feet where I could see him through the mirror and he always counted down the time for each segment letting me know when it was almost over. The only two times I had difficulty was once when the noise sounded like some sort of sonar ping and I began imagining myself as a torpedo. This brought about giggles and I worried if I didn't stop, I would move and the test would have to begin anew. The second time, was near the end. Of course I would suddenly need to use the restroom! Once they have you positioned they want you to stay that way so stopping for a bathroom break is not really feasible. Thankfully, the next run was only 4 minutes and then the whole thing was over. I was so relaxed in fact that in the middle I almost fell asleep.

Since this time, I have had two other MRI's and am now feeling like a vet. I know to ask for sedation beforehand, and Mark knows to rub my feet and count down the clock for me. I know what to expect, how long it will be and although I am still claustrophobic, I have at least been able to make the experience almost comfortable. Besides, how better to get as foot massage from your husband?

This is about where my diagnostic story ends and my first book, Coffee in the Cereal: The First Year with Multiple Sclerosis begins. I did make it through the second spinal tap and knew when I got home to lay flat. I did get the spinal headache again but it was nothing that required a trip to the hospital, just bed rest and loads of Motrin. After the MRI, and second spinal tap,

I went in to get the results. Instead, my neurologist when look-ing down at my file and results must have forgotten I had not yet been given a final diagnosis, and asked the famous ques-tion:

"So, what are you taking for your MS?"

Chapter II

Cognitive Shifts

Bats in the Belfry

Cognitive problems. Most people with MS experience this everyday. For quite some time, in fact, doctors did not believe that MS effected the brain in this way. Thankfully for those of us with MS, they've changed their minds. Cognitive problems are now addressed at seminars, in medical journals and current MS books.

After I developed Multiple Sclerosis, my mind changed too. Not just about whether or not wearing high heels was an attempt at breaking my neck either. At times, my thoughts became fuzzy and difficult. Sometimes I could even get myself lost in my house or forget simple words. Of course, now after five years, I know where the kitchen is and I either call things by their appropriate name or make up for my word-loss with "thingy." When faced with bills or applications, I was often reduced to frustrated tears. Now, I only cry when I see the amount owed. Even though living with these cognitive problems can be rough and sometimes very depressing, there are ways to adapt.

The first thing I learned to do was laugh. Okay, it was more like the third thing after buying various timers and obsessively taking notes to not forget things. But after that I learned to laugh. Because out of all my symptoms, my cognitive screw-ups are the easiest to laugh at. Of course, my husband, Mark doesn't think the melting of our spatula was funny, but it does look rather abstract and amusing these days as it hangs on our wall. Realizing that on bad days you can't be trusted to cook for your kids, can be depressing. But noticing that your son would rather have cereal with milk in it, as opposed to the coffee you just poured in, can be seen as another failing or down right funny. I chose funny. Especially when the milk was still sitting in the cupboard next to the cereal. How else could I get by if I did not learn to laugh at myself?

One day while on the way to see my neurologist, I became very hot and thirsty. As we entered the building, my husband noticed that I was avidly searching for something.

"What are you looking for, Hon?" he asked leading me towards the elevator.

"I'm looking for a sprinkler," I replied matter-of-factly. I did not notice my husband's eyebrows shoot up in confusion.

"Why?" he asked calmly.

"Because I'm thirsty. You'd think they had sprinklers in an office building so someone could get a drink of water," I replied still looking around. My husband only smiled to himself and made an affirmative noise by humming. When we reached the elevator, I sighed deeply realizing I would not find what I was looking for. As we stepped in, I huffed loudly, "I can't believe they don't have any sprinklers in here!"

As the doors to the elevator began to close, my brain suddenly repeated the last few sentences in my head. I knew something was wrong with them. There was a word out of place. My husband remained silent beside me as if nothing out the ordinary had happened. When the doors opened again, it was as if my brain had opened it's own doors. The realization of what I had been saying swept through me and I began to giggle.

"DRINKING FOUNTAIN!" I shouted slapping my hand to my forehead. I looked at my husband and started to laugh. "That whole time I said I was looking for a sprinkler I had meant drinking fountain. Wow that was weird!" I stepped out of the elevator with my husband behind me. I paused and looked over my shoulder at my mate. "Why didn't you correct me? You didn't say a word!"

He simply smiled and placed an arm about my waist smiling. "I knew what you meant. Besides, they both give out water. It made sense."

The trouble with word-finding has become increasingly diffi- cult over the past few years. Everyone can get a bit jumbled in times of stress but for those of us with MS, this cognitive issue can get worse along with the progression of the disease. Many articles offer the advice to slow-down and wait for the words to come. In my experience this only works if I am talking to an- other MSer or someone who has an understanding of what I am doing. Otherwise people look at you funny as you stand there with your eyes focused on the ceiling, waiting for lighten- ing to strike your brain. Or, more often, they will finish your sentences for you and run away without a complete under- standing of what you were trying to say in the first place. So the next thing I learned to do after laughing was relaxing. But not relaxing and waiting for a word, instead just letting it all go.

Once I learned to laugh and relax, it didn't bother me that I call my cats chickens sometimes or could not remember the dog's name. In fact, my son burst out laughing when Mommy called the dog "who-sit." I don't cry when I can't concentrate on my favorite book long enough to read a few pages. I don't scream when I found I've put the mobile phone in the freezer. Although it is frightening when you're getting a TV dinner and suddenly the frozen chicken starts vibrating and singing the Cingular tune. It no longer upsets me that my husband refers to me as "the only woman who can stand in the shampoo aisle for twenty minutes reading the back of one bottle." (By the way, have you ever read those things? Do you realize what you're putting in your hair? Herbal my a**!)I just laugh. I shake my head, smile and remember the words of a wise man that counseled me once:

"If you try to battle and beat down your MS, every time you will lose. But if you accept it as part of yourself and work with it, you will find yourself less lost, angry, and tired."

Okay. This was probably as close as I ever came to becoming one with MS, I'll admit it. But he had a point. Why waste any-more time crying, when I could be laughing? Why frustrate myself with the grocery shopping when my husband could do it, and I could commune with a bottle of strawberry scented Suave? Why tense up and break down when I could not re-member my son's birth-date when instead, I could take a deep breath, relax my shoulders and know it would come if I just became still.

When I find myself battling with cognitive problems and be-coming upset, I try to remember this: Stillness and laughter. If I go with the flow of the river, I will be fine. If I panic and fight the current, I will only be sucked under. I cannot change the course of this river and I cannot change how fast or slow the current moves, but I can choose to relax. I can choose to be tickled by the water rushing around me. Okay enough river comparisons. There are days when cognitive problems cripple me and I do get angry and discouraged. No one can be ac-cepting and cheery all the time. There are times when I laugh but I do it through my tears. But there are also times when that laughter is honest and healing. So why not try it?

MS Dialect
(Or a lesson in the proper use of "thingy")

I cannot pinpoint the exact time that thingy became part of my MS vocabulary, but I do know that after five years, it is now a common part of my speech. Thingy, also known as thingamabob or thingamajig, and is any item for which I have forgotten the proper English name. Now everyone occasionally says "get me that thingy," or "hand me that whatsit," especially as they near old age, but as an MSer with cognitive problems I can assure you that I use this word more often.

Cognitive difficulties in MS are not uncommon and I would hazard a guess that after fatigue they are the second most common invisible symptom in MS. Among cognitive difficulties in MS are memory loss, attention span deficits, and problems with word-finding. Word-finding trouble is what originally birthed my excessive use of the word "thingy." For some reason, probably being a mother, and using baby talk, I feel compelled to call it a thingy and not a thing. Just like it's a blanky, wipey, and ducky.

My use of this word has progressed along with my MS. In the beginning, it was only used sparingly at times when I was overtired or stressed. During these instances my brain, like a computer low on memory, would save space and energy by only allowing access to only certain files. The rest of my system was temporarily off-line, so to speak. No pun intended.

While many board games are played by the player not being allowed to use specific words, an average person has a vast store of synonyms that can be used at any time when another word has been eliminated from their vocabulary. For instance, if the game called for a person to get a teammate to say blueberry, but they cannot use the words "blue" or "berry," they could say something like "small round fruit." I would say "blue thingies" and lose the game.

Here is an example of a common occurrence. I'm in the living room and I have left my soda in the kitchen. I want to ask Mark to retrieve the soda from the counter. I give myself points for even remembering where I left the soda in the first place. That is a rare day indeed. But unable to remember the words "kitchen counter," I end up saying something like this: "Babe, could you get me the drink I left on the thingy?"

"Where?" Mark has learned that if he could just get a better sense of the location, he might find the item.

Realizing my words did not aptly describe what I want, I attempt to restate my request adding in a directional phrase while pointing, "It's on the thingy in the room out there where we put the stuff." Now Mark heads for the kitchen and I figure we had victory on our hands. Until he continues through the kitchen and into our bedroom figuring that this is where we put all the stuff. Seeing his mistake, I now shout, "The Soda is on the flat thing in there!" However, I do not realize that while I am pointing in the kitchen, Mark is in the bedroom and cannot see my fingers. You'd think men could get eyes in the backs of their heads like most women have. So now he is wandering around the bedroom lost.

"Which flat thing?"

"Not in there. In THERE!" I holler.

"What? The bathroom?" By now I have my head buried in the couch cushions groaning. Why couldn't he figure this out? Why can't the spouses of disabled people come with remote controls so you can propel them in the direction you need? At this point, you must be wondering why I did not get off my butt and go get the soda. Well, because it had now become a proving point. I had to prove I could adequately get him to find the drink without the ability to talk correctly. Or maybe I was just having too much fun watching him wander throughout the house confused.

"Not the bathroom, out here!" I call again. Mark comes stomping back out of the bedroom.

"Well if it's in there with you, why did you send me to another room?" Mark asked moving through the kitchen.

"Stop right there! It's in there!" I was now waving my hands and pointing. Mark looked down to his right at the soda on the kitchen counter. Of course he could not resist educating me on the correct words.

"Oh! You meant kitchen counter," he remarked grabbing it and bringing it to me.

"Yes, I know." When he turned back into the kitchen I made faces at him. Childish, maybe, stress relieving? Totally.

As the years have gone by and my MS has progressed, "thingy" became a catch-all term used not only in times of stress or fatigue. "It's on the thingy in there" became a common statement around the house.

One day while cooking, I found I needed a spatula but could not remember the name. I often get worse off when cooking because I am using so much of my concentration on not burning things. I was adding more cheese to my breakfast omelet when Mark asked if I needed anything. He tends to hover when I am using the stove. I have since my diagnosis killed one stove, one pot, and various plastic utensils.

"Yes I need the thingy in the drawer," I replied, thankful that he could grab the spatula while I tended to the veggies going into the omelet.

"Which thingy is it, Love?"

"The flat one."

"The flat thingy or the flat drawer?" he asked, laughing. The eggs were congealing faster and I waved the whisk at him spraying goopy egg in his direction.

"Drawer number two," I replied pointing with the whisk. He pulled open the drawer and stared into it.

"Um Hon, what are you cooking?"

"Eggs."

"Would it be a spatula that you need?"

"Smart ass. If I'm threatening you with the whisk and cooking the eggs what else would I need? Hurry, the eggs are burning."

"Well, why didn't you get the spatula then?" There he went using the word repeatedly as if that would help next time.

"Because you asked if I needed anything!"

While "thingy" was originally the only word I used, after five years with MS, I know commonly useful sentences involving no real words whatsoever. What has always puzzled Mark is that I would rather give out longer requests than to take a deep breath and quietly wait for the word to come to me. This definitely does not work when the eggs are burning. In this day and age when everything is accomplished by multi-tasking at a frantic pace, it seems only natural that I would rather shout over 20 words and five sentences with full arm waving and finger pointing to get my point across, than wait. The latest hypothesis Mark has for my strange behavior is that I have entered in a full on battle with my brain. He believes that I think if I just keep talking long enough, while waving my arms, either the word will be forced out or I'll achieve lift off. Being the world's first flying woman, I could hire someone to talk for me. Also, after five years Mark has become very fluent in Thingy.

Although I have tried daily doses of Gingko Biloba and Provigil to increase brainpower and ward off fatigue, there is no medication as of yet that can help with the word-finding. It seems unfortunate that despite all the recent progress in the study of Multiple Sclerosis, that this part of cognitive difficulty has not been given more attention. Then again it would make sense that they are more interested in a cure or dealing with major symptoms like fatigue and muscle weakness than to deal with a poor woman's inability to say "kitchen counter."

I am not the only patient affected daily by this difficulty but it appears to be not a significant enough symptom to matter. Most doctors want to focus on symptoms which interfere heavily with a patient's quality of life and to them calling, the refrigerator "the cold thingy with food" is not sufficient interference. In fact I would bet they find it down right amusing.

I often wonder about the spouses and family members though, whom run about the house trying to solve the vague thingy quest. Is it fair to them? Of course not, but it IS amusing for the MSer. Honestly we need more reasons to be amused by our own flaws. It is very depressing for me to find myself in a conversation with another professional, trying desperately to sound intelligent and together, and coming off sounding either slow or just plain odd. So if watching my husband or son run around the house trying to find the "thingy" can point out the humorous side to an otherwise frustrating and depressing cognitive

Chapter 2

issue, then so be it!

Now go get me that thingy over there.

Slur-py: MS & Speech

Speech is one of the first things that we recognize in children as a great step towards becoming an adult. It is also occasionally one of the first symptoms for people with MS who are effected more cognitively than physically. At the time in our life when we need most to communicate about our feelings and needs, our brain cuts off its long term relationship with our mouth. I have tried repeatedly to get these two back together but have only succeeded in a rocky relationship that quits half the time. Yet it amazes me that when I feel I am speaking with the proficiency of a drooling two-year old, no-one seems to notice. (Except the two-year olds.)

I am beginning to believe that Multiple Sclerosis is not only unpredictable, but that it has a very sick sense of humor. On days when I am proud of myself for appearing only half psychotic, my family tells me that my speech is slurred. I do not hear this; in fact I think my speech has been clearer than ever. Yet when I feel I am struggling to get words out and my mind feels like it is having some sort of syllable traffic jam, people tell me that they notice nothing. To make things worse, when I apologize for this jolted speech they reply, "Why, your speech is much clearer than normal!" These people should know that there are rules about teasing the crazy people.

Now either my family is playing a nasty trick on me, and considering the fact that my family's jokes range from perverse to little rubber frogs wrapped as Christmas gifts, this IS possible. Or this feeling of an inability to speak is another one of those brilliantly mischievous and invisible symptoms of MS. When researching this odd occurrence online, I found that the slurring of speech is technically referred to as "dysarthria." Saying

51

this word alone would make a person slur. "Doctor, I have dysssarthhria."

Dysarthria is difficult, poorly articulated speech. Looking at this definition I resigned to diagnose all workers of a fast food drive-thru with dysarthria. I always knew it wasn't MY hearing! I also vowed to add dysarthria to my list of big words as it sounded much more educated than "slurred speech." I have wondered if my doctor even used this word.

On further examination I found that this horrible condition can be caused by alcohol, badly fitted dentures, or (big surprise) a degenerative neurological disorder. Hmm. Now my family and friends would not believe the denture excuse for one minute. Blaming it on alcohol would not be prudent when at the grocery store at 10:00 a.m., especially if just happened to run into my son's school teacher or anyone else I know. I never imagined that alcohol, dentures, and a neurological disorder could be put into the same medical arena. This then led me to wonder about those with MS who drink and also have dentures. How do they know if it is dysarthria or their teeth?

To make things more complicated, as I read on another word flashed across the screen. Another word that when pronounced, would cause anyone to slur. Aphasia. How is that pronounced anyhow? Af-asia? That sounds like some old historical term for post Asia. "Af-Asia," after Asia. But I digress. Aphasia is: impaired expression or comprehension of the spoken or written word, but it has the common courtesy to go away after a period. The only thing I know that goes away after a period is bloating. Hmmm, I wondered. When I have speech attacks, does this mean it's Dysarthria or Aphasia? I glanced over the causes for Aphasia and accidentally snorted my soda. Head trauma, stroke, and Alzheimer's. I'd rather be drunk with bad dentures. Make that into a bumper sticker and put it on your car.

This still did not explain the fact that when I slurred I did not notice it and when I felt I was stuttering no-one heard it. Nevertheless, after blowing my nose and cleaning up the soda, it dawned on me. Drunk people believe their speech is clear and I know my Grandpa never seemed to realize his dentures where sticking out of his mouth. And boy did that lead to some horrible nightmares. Nothing worse than a bushy eye-browed old man with his teeth hanging out chasing you down a hall.

Now I could begin to grasp the idea that although I did not hear it, it could still be going on. This left me to look for a cure. Surely there was a way to get my tongue back in order. For dysarthria, slurring, the suggested cure was "speaking slowly and using hand gestures." I pictured myself giving orders to my pharmacist while slowly speaking and waving my hands. I was pretty sure it wouldn't go over well, although he might slip an extra bottle of pills into my order. Then this report stated that family and friends needed to give me, "the afflicted person," time enough to express myself. Yeah, right. My son is really going to stand around while Mommy figures out how to say "clean your room" slowly and while pantomiming sweeping. He might giggle for a moment, but he wouldn't be around for me to finish.

To cure Aphasia, the family is urged to give the person reminders when they slip up, such as why the house smells like smoke and they have a string on their finger. It follows by saying that for both afflictions a "calm environment where external stimuli is kept to a minimum is extremely important." A calm environment. I was equally sure that my family was not going to appreciate my decision to move to the mountains and bury myself in a hole, because that is about where I'd need to go to get calmness in my life. Moreover, how can a person exist without external stimuli and in the case of a MSer external stimuli is rarely at a minimum! The air on our skin can be disrupting external stimuli.

So waving my arms and demanding serenity while stress relieving for me, was still not going to solve any speech problems. After years of living with MS in which my cognitive abilities have only gone downhill, I will admit to frantic hand motions and arm waving. This is usually accompanied by my attempts to describe things without adjectives because I have suddenly forgotten words. More on that later.

As for the slurring and stuttering, they seem to go hand in hand. While they have not progressed as my other speech difficulties have, they pop up in times of relapse or heavy stress, and the occasional holiday gathering after one too many eggnogs sans the egg. I have not found a cure for this nor do people seem to notice unless I think I'm fine. So the best way I have found to deal with this type of speech problem is to simply wait and see. If someone brings up the slur, I tell them all about Multiple Sclerosis. If they don't and look at me funny, I tell them all about my MS, because lord knows what they're really thinking. But if I feel out of place with my tongue yet no one is looking at me strangely nor approaching me with sign language thinking I have a hearing problem, I just go about my day. Waving my arms, using hand signals, and swearing I'm drunk. Or wearing dentures.

The Notebook Saga. (MS OCD)

MS is full of diversity, not only from person to person but in each body. One day, it's pins and needles up your leg and the next, you can't pee. For those who aren't affected so greatly, it's one day you're tired and the next you're well- not? We of course do this on purpose to make our health care professionals and family members go nuts. I like to think my body has its own union that can go on strike at any time for absolutely no reason. This inability to predict anything has not led me into the graceful ability to "go with the flow," but instead has spawned a nasty controlling streak in me.

I don't think people suddenly develop obsessive compulsive disorder (OCD) in their late 20's, so that has lead me to the conclusion that my new found penchant for obsessively taking notes and making lists is a compensation for my MS. While I do have to admit to being a neurotic worrywart before my diagnosis, in the last five years I have turned into a completely new breed of neurotic worry-wart. You could say I've moved from little worried dog to obsessive herding dog status. If you don't know dogs, just trust me. There is a big difference between the neuroses of a poodle "Who's at the door?" and a border collie "Who's at the door? Where is my owner going? What is the kid doing? Where is the cat going? Was that a fly? Who's at the door?"

Controlling everything in Multiple Sclerosis is impossible. Therefore, I began to control as much of everything else as possible. I couldn't seem to keep my memory in hand so I controlled the problem by writing everything down. At first I tried calendars making sure I wrote every appointment down on the calendar near the phone as soon as I got it. This way I would never again miss an appointment. This only worked if I looked at the calendar on the day of the appointment. So I got three calendars. One calendar for by the phone, one near my computer, and another on the fridge. This still only worked if I looked at the calendar, but only if I had written the appointment or reminder on the calendars themselves. It also helps to look at the correct day! Oftentimes, I looked at the wrong week and thought, "Oh, good! My appointment isn't until next week," when actually it was that day. When I missed an appointment not because I hadn't looked at the calendar, but because it simply didn't register that what was written needed to be done THAT day, I moved on to sticky notes.

Sticky notes initially were very useful for instant reminders. I would stick them on the TV, the monitor of my computer, the mirror, any place I thought I would look in order to remind me of important dates, shows, etc. Then came the problem. They wouldn't stay stuck. At first, I thought I had simply bought cheap sticky notes, so I went to the store and bought the most expensive sticky notes I could find. They still didn't stick. Sure sometimes they can remain in place for 24 hours, but beyond that the shelf life of a once stuck sticky note, is pretty dismal. They begin to slide, curl, or simply commit suicide, and oftentimes within the first 30 seconds. I began to wonder if the person that created sticky notes was not some sadistic madman running through a factory shouting, "Then they'll fall of and the people will replace the note with another sticky note, which will fall off! Then they'll use more and more and more until they have to buy MORE sticky notes! Muhahahahaha!"

I got desperate. I began scotch-taping my "sticky" notes to things. I was determined to not give in to needless spending of my family's funds for more sticky notes. Two problems arose. The tape didn't stick or it didn't come off. I came to the conclusion at this point that all inventors of any kind of adhesive tape or paper with adhesive were evil. The only person you could count on, who must have had proper up bringing, was Mr. Elmer.

His glue always worked. Needless to say my husband was not about to allow me to Elmer my sticky notes to the TV, that by the way holds sticky notes much better after being dusted, so I resigned myself to sticky notes on plastics -like the side of my monitor, and paper.

After securing the wealth of the sticky note factory for at least a few months, I developed a new and lasting way of keeping track of every appointment. I bought a notebook. Not some fancy organizer just a plain spiral ring notebook. When I was given the appointment, I wrote it on a note pad and then, if I remembered, I wrote it on the three calendars. With my cognitive difficulties and ways of remembering things wrong or not at all, I always asked the receptionist to read the appointment back to me and then insisted that she listen while read it back to her. Because more than once I'd say "the 24th," and write "the 27th." This way, when I read back exactly what I'd written she could correct me and I could snap, "Well, why didn't you say that in the first place?"

As time went by, I began to rely more on the notebook and one calendar than all Three. Then it was down to only the notebook. It now held all important family information and I carried it with me everywhere. I knew at all times where the notebook was. It went with me in the car and came on outings with me. I took it everywhere. And then my husband used it and it was gone.

Now men carry the "y" gene. It's what makes them men. Okay it takes a lot more than a gene to make a man a man, but scientifically speaking it's that one gene. What most people don't know, but women have suspected since the beginning of time, is that men are also afflicted with a genetic disorder that causes them to make things disappear. At first, this disorder presents itself in the male only losing his own things. This is now evident in my seven year-old-son, who without my help, would go to school barefoot and with no underwear, because he can't find them. Of course, they are right there staring at him from the underwear drawer.

This disorder, I've come to believe, is some sort of vision discrepancy because most often the item is sitting in plain sight with the male circling around it. I also suspect that vision is not the only sense impaired, for if the item is not in plain sight, it is usually in the most logical place, but men can't seem to grasp this concept either. Asking, "Where did you have it last?" is about as successful with most men as asking, "Is my butt big?" They never give satisfactory answers. Also, as the male grows so does this condition. In later years, he becomes infectious, tainting not only his own property but also whatever else he touches. Thus, when Mark used the notebook, it disappeared.

At first being the female, and the antidote to male-pattern blindness, I was confident that I would find the notebook. But I didn't. As I rummaged through his desk and then did a once over glance at every flat surface in the house, I began to lose my composure. The whole house became a possible hiding place. Having found his keys once on top of the refrigerator and his wallet under the bathtub, I knew I had an adventure ahead of me. But I didn't want a challenge this time. I wanted the notebook back safe and sound. I wasn't gloating in my female ability to locate items but instead was beginning to add up the percentage of times items had been lost forever. Tearing apart the house, some heavy stress began to set in. I had not been writing anything on the calendars. The notebook held not only appointments, but also phone numbers I'd never put in my Rolodex and computations of how much each bill would be. Everything was in that notebook, and now he'd touched it!

Days went by with no sight of the notebook and numerous arguments about how Mark could lose such an important item. To him, it had only been something to write on while he was on the phone. He had no attachment to it, and did not see why the loss of it was causing such a stir. I contemplated banishing him from the bedroom until he found it. While Mark is often so understanding of my condition that people wish to nominate him for sainthood, there are times when he is just a man.

Around day five of the missing notebook I was tearing through the laundry room when yet again Mark remarked casually that, "It would turn up." I began by trying to explain, for the fortieth time, how important the item was, and finished by yelling and throwing clothes at him while I burst into frustrated tears. Most people might think that this reaction was over the top. But this notebook had become my cognitive crutch. In a good way. I knew I had no control over how my MS was going to effect my body but I did have control over how I compensated with what it gave me. The notebook was my compensation for cognitive problems. Without it, I was lost and frankly I didn't like the helpless feeling.

Cognitive difficulties, including memory problems, had been one of the first symptoms of my MS and also the hardest to explain to people. When a healthy looking 28-year-old misses a birthday or an appointment with the explanation of "I forgot," most people assume I am simply selfish and lazy. In those five days, I knew that I was going to forget things and wondered how many health professionals and friends I was going to piss off because of something I had forgotten. I lay awake at night wracking my brain trying to remember what had been in the book and only succeeded in getting the new Mazda commercial with a song that said "zoom zoom zoom" stuck in my head.

Eventually I gave up and bought another notebook. Staring at the blank pages, I felt sick. I didn't have the number to my son's school. I didn't know when my next appointment with the neurologist was or if I had missed it. And I knew I had a lot of work ahead of me to catch up. At this point I could barely look at Mark. He spent most of those days avoiding me or talking to me in soft tones, often used when he feels I am likely to be irrational and throw things. I rarely throw things. If I do, I only use cloth and pillows. You know, healthy expressions of un-controllable rage.

Thus began the task of calling various doctors' offices to find out what I had missed or what was coming up. Then it was time to look up the phone number for my son's school, call my mother for birth dates, and spend hours trying to fill the new notebook with whatever pertinent information I could recall being in the previous book. It was on this day that Mark went over to his parent's house to do some car work. They only live a few blocks away and we visit them often. Mark and his father work together and so it is not uncommon for them to be driving back and forth to each other's home. I was about two hours in to re-filling the book when Mark came home. He entered the bedroom, where my desk and computer are, and approached me with a strange look on his face and his hands behind his back. I finished my phone conversation with my mother and looked at him.

"What is it?" Mark brought a hand from behind his back and held out my old notebook.

"Apparently, I left it at Dad's," he murmured. The next hand came out from behind his back and handed me a bouquet of flowers. "I'm sorry this happened." I snatched both items and looked at him with confusion.

"But we called them and asked if it was there. They said no."

"Yes. Well, Dad had written some messages down on it and it was by their phone until Mom noticed that it was not theirs," Mark smiled. I snorted.

"So you stole my notebook to write down messages, then you took it to your dad's where he stole it from you, to write down messages?" I shook my head in amazement.

"It appears that is what happened."

"And of course it was a woman who noticed the notebook was misplaced." I pointed out.

"Yes, Hon. As soon as Mom saw your handwriting she knew it was the one you had been looking for. She demanded I stop working on the cars and bring it back immediately."

"Good for her," I muttered, smelling the flowers.

"It seems Mom has her own notebook by the phone as well," Mark mentioned over his shoulder as he went to get a vase for the bouquet.

"Oh really? Then why was your Dad using mine?" I called out. Mark laughed.

"Because he'd lost hers."

In the end we both apologized to each other. Me for being such a royal pain when I had lost the notebook and Mark for not understanding how important it was for my cognitive sanity to keep my things in their place. After seeing how much anguish I went through, he recognized how important some compensation for my MS had become. I would like to say that since then he has never misplaced another of my notebooks, but that would be a lie. I now carry an average of three notebooks and try to keep him in a supply of blank cheap pads to write on. I also now have a big 60 day calendar that is erasable on the kitchen wall. No one can miss it, not even an MSer with memory problems.

And Then You Forget

It was summer, and about three years after my diagnosis. I had learned to not hyper focus on every little problem as being caused by my MS. I had come to grips with the concept that maybe remission in my case meant accepting a form of "this is as good as it gets," instead of waiting to go back to Pre-MS Lorna. (This is different from PMS-Lorna.) I'd quit reading all the MS books and magazine articles and had basically adopted a "Yeah. I have MS, and my cat has six toes, so what?" attitude. But there are still times when this type of coping can be hazardous to my health.

One day somewhere in the middle of summer, I began to feel crappy. I was tired most of the day, taking extra naps, and generally feeling under the weather. When my legs began to get achy and I kept moving them to try to get them comfortable, I assumed I had the flu. I sat on my bed, which is where our family spends the most time acting like Romans by lounging about eating and watching gladiator programs on the Discovery channel, with my legs shifting. It was not a violent thrashing, but a sort of rubbing them, crossing and uncrossing my ankles and generally feeling unable to get comfortable. My husband, Mark noted this. When he asked, I told him I had a bug. Life went on as normal the way it does when Mommy is not feeling well.

After about four days of lying about nothing had let up. I felt worse. There was nothing major happening that would make me suspect MS. Nothing was numb or leaking, so I still figured I had a virus of some sort. I just felt blah. I knew my extra napping and general listless attitude was not depression because at the time I was taking enough Zoloft to make Van

Gogh think happy thoughts. I never pondered MS, because it simply didn't seem fitting. Or maybe I was just being a dunce.

The next summer morning, I forced myself out of bed and began doing household chores. I sorted the laundry and drug the baskets out to the laundry room. Mark barely raised an eyebrow when he saw me kicking the basket across the kitchen and then dragging it out the door. He knew I hated asking for help and must have been able to tell by the set of my jaw or the steel in my eyes that I was determined to get things done. So he went out to the shop to work and left me to finish proving that I could alleviate flu with serious housework.

I began by washing the whites in the usual mix of hot water and bleach, and then moved into the kitchen to start the dishwasher. I sprinkled the powder in, shut the door, and headed to the bathroom because everyone knows you can kick the flu by scrubbing a claw-footed bathtub while inhaling noxious fumes. After scrubbing the stains for awhile, I remembered to check on the laundry. By this point, the whites were done washing and I moved the load into the dryer not noticing the pink spots all over the socks and the red shirt that had caused them. I started the next load of wash and meandered back into the kitchen. I wasn't worried about my cognitive abilities, because when I am at my cognitive worst, I am also usually blissfully unaware of how daft I'm being. It's like grandma talking about her safe driving skills as she takes the wrong exit at 80 m.p.h.

In the kitchen, I decided to make some tea and stopped the dishwasher mid-cycle to pull out a mug. I then set the kettle on the stove. Feeling very proud of myself, I went back to the bathroom where I filled the tub with warm water and bleach to let it soak, before I rinsed it down again. I then finished wiping down the bathroom counters, scrubbing the toilet and washing the mirrors. At this point I began to feel tired and went back into the kitchen to grab a snack. The dishwasher was not making any noise, so figuring the cycle was done, I emptied it. I had taught myself not to do any serious cooking without Mark in the house, so I popped a corndog in the microwave and went back out to check on the whites, promptly forgetting the corndog. The whites were finished, so I piled them into a small basket and headed for the bedroom where I could stretch out and fold clothes while watching TV.

I dumped the whites on the bed and flopped down to enjoy my TV. Sometime during the movie, and my folding, the tea pot must have begun to boil. But because I had not closed the spout on the kettle, it was not whistling loudly to let me know the water was done. Instead the boiling water began shooting from the spout in little spurts on to the stove creating a hissing noise.

Happily folding my husbands pink socks (Because it was of course his fault there was a red shirt in with the whites, although he never sorts the laundry), a quiet hissing noise began to come from the kitchen. Did I run in remembering my tea water? No. It would have whistled if it were the tea pot. Instead, I turned up the TV because I knew it must be my son's video game making too much noise. Now did my son notice the noise? Yes. But he figured mom knew what she was doing and either wanted it that way or would be in to fix it momentarily.

Instead it was Mark, coming back in from a day's work in the shop, who came to the rescue of the tea pot before the water had boiled away and the pot itself began to burn. It was Mark who noticed the "washed" and put away glasses that had suspicious amounts of dish powder attached to them. My husband and often my savior had slipped into the bedroom to find me dead asleep amongst the pink laundry half folded with the TV on. When I came out of my coma-like stupor, I found him sitting on the bed reading a book.

"Hey, Hon. How are you feeling?" He was using that sweet,

64

hushed tone. The one you use with sick people and wild animals. I immediately got suspicious. I hadn't been feeling well for days and had not received the sympathetic tone yet.

"What's wrong?" I asked pushing up into a sitting position and trying to disentangle myself from a shirt that looked tie-died by Barney. I was amazed at how disoriented I felt, like a person coming out from under anesthesia.

"You were making some tea?" he asked gently.

"Oh damn!" I threw back the sheet I had draped over myself, knocking some spotted underwear to the floor and made to get out of bed but Mark laid a hand on my ankle.

"I already turned it off."

"God. I cannot believe I forgot that. I must have drifted off while I was folding the laundry."

"And the bathtub?" There was the tone again. Soft and gentle.

"What about it? I cleaned it."

"There is bleach in the tub still."

"Oh, crap. I filled it up with hot water and bleach to let it soak and forgot to drain it.

"When was that?" I looked over at the clock. 4:00 p.m. Had I slept that long? I had filled the tub at around noon.

"It was a bit ago," I remarked, hedging a direct answer. Mark gave me a look. I squirmed and played with a pair of pink socks.

"So what happened with the laundry?" Mark nodded to the socks.

"Red shirt."

"And the dishes?"

Now I got defensive. I had done nothing wrong with the dishes. "I washed them and put them away!" Somehow Mark materialized a glass spotted with dish powder crystals. My shoulders sagged. "That's why they finished so fast." Mark now looked somewhere between pity and laughter. I could tell he was waiting for me. Waiting to see if I would connect the dots and also waiting to see how I would react to it. Instead I got out of bed and slipped on my flip-fops, ignoring the heavy urge to go back to sleep. "Maybe I have A.D.D.," I snapped.

"Maybe you have MS," Mark replied. I shot him an irritated look.

"Excuse me?"

"Babe, you're doing it again."

"Doing what?" I grumbled, sitting back on the bed.

"Forgetting your limitations and ignoring your symptoms."

"What symptoms? My eye is fine. I'm walking and I don't have vertigo."

"What about debilitating fatigue, feeling in a fog, and restless leg syndrome?" Mark reached for my hand. "Let's not forget cognitive problems."

"Oh, ha ha. And don't forget cognitive problems," I repeated.

"No pun intended," he remarked trying not to laugh. "Only you would talk like that."

"Sure. You don't have a teasing bone in your body." I removed his hand and crossed my arms, leaning back against the pillows. Not because I was tired but because it felt good. Who was I kidding? I was exhausted. "The red shirt could happen to anyone. Same goes for the tub and the dishwasher. The tea pot as well." Mark sighed and shook his head.

"Yes. But the reason we have a tea pot made of industrial strength steel is because you have a penchant for randomly testing the melting points of cookware," he laughed and I fought to not giggle with him.

"That only counts for plastics!" Mark leveled his gaze at me. "Okay and spaghetti pots." Still he stared. "All right and now tea kettles."

"Now tea pots? Have you forgotten how many incidents we've had in the last three years? What about the time we had the herb garden?"

"What does our herb garden have to do with the teapot?" I snuggled more against the pillows and kept my hands out of his reach. I didn't feel like admitting he was right and I didn't like where he was going with the topic. No one likes hearing that they can't be trusted to cook and clean for their family. Then again, no more cooking and cleaning for the family sounded heavenly.

"You put the lavender in a pot with hot water to simmer and make the house smell good."

"Oh." I began to remember.

"And the water boiled away."

"Yep."

"And the lavender stuck to the bottom of the pot."

"Yes, but I rescued it before it burned!" I said triumphantly.

"But it was congealed mass of gunk! That could have burned."

"Yes, but a nice smelling congealed mass. That didn't burn."

"Okay I'll give you that, but that is not my point." Uh-oh.

"So your point is?"

"Cognitive problems." Mark handed me the book he'd been reading. I didn't look at it.

"Well yes cognitive problems can interfere with speech, performance IQ, and finding words."

"And memory, Hon. It has to be your MS." I finally looked down at the book on the bed. The book was: Multiple Sclerosis A Guide for Families by Rosalind Kalb. It was a book I had not touched since I first read it after my diagnosis. It was opened to a page and Mark had underlined a passage reading: "Well intentioned family and friends will say things like 'Oh, I forget appointments too that happens to everybody.' Such reassurances tend to invalidate what is a very real set of problems based on a specific neurologic disease" (p. 25). I flipped back a couple of pages and stared in awe as it listed memory and then attention and concentration as the top examples of cognitive impairment. I looked up at Mark who still had that sappy sympathetic look on his face. I loved him for recognizing the symptoms and hated him for being right. He's a bear to live with when he's right. I couldn't give him the upper hand. I was not going to burst into tears over the fact that my brain was yet again showing its holes and that I was not capable of being supermom multitasking my way through life. I would not cry this time! Instead, I shrugged my shoulders and smiled.

"This section on cognitive impairment is very interesting. How nice of you to point it out." Mark looked nervous. He loved being right but he knew I hated being wrong.

"You're not upset? I'm sorry I had to point this out and I tried to be as gentle as possible-"

"You were perfect and I love you for it. I'm glad you brought this to my attention." I gave him a huge hug and a quick peck on the cheek before forcing myself off the bed again and making my way to the kitchen to make yet another pot of water for tea. Mark followed.

"You're not angry?"

"Nope."

"Not even a little bit upset about having to face your limitations?"

"Not at all," I replied cheerfully as I put the kettle back on. Mark leaned against the counter and shook his head.

"All right. I give. Why are you not upset?" I turned and gave him a Cheshire cat grin and giggled.

"Because tomorrow, I'll forget this ever happened."

* * * * * *

But I did remember my books. When times came that I felt I was not meeting my supermom quota or I just felt off, it was helpful to go back to the beginning. Back to my books on MS and sometimes back to my own writings and postings on MS MOMS. These often helped "remind" me of issues such as cognitive problems that I had faced in the past and simply forgot. I may not always remember the tea and have issues with appointments, but at least I knew how to find help. If I could just remember to look for it.

REFERENCE

Kalb, Rosalind C., PhD. 1998. *Multiple Sclerosis: A Guide for Families.*
     New York: Demos Vermande.

CHAPTER III

FLARE-UPS
AND
OTHER NEUROSES

D.O.S

Fatigue. Otherwise known as the overwhelming, wow the wooden floor isn't that hard, dust bunnies taste good, oh there's my earring!, flat on your belly lifelessness. Do you find yourself leaning on things more than standing? Are you completely at ease with lowering yourself to the floor in a bookstore to rest? Do you let yourself be decorated like a Christmas tree by your nieces and nephews because you couldn't move if you wanted to? Then you know what it is like to battle MS fatigue! According to the National Multiple Sclerosis Society, fatigue affects around 80% of people with MS. The fact that a large number of the MS population is women with children may or may not be the reason we're always so damned exhausted.

The way most people with MS deal with fatigue is with moderation and sometimes with medication. Although many advances have been made in medications that slow the progression of MS, there is still not much to be offered in medications for fatigue. Most medications for fatigue are controlled substances, for example Cylert. Or they can be heavy on side-effects, like Amantadine. Provigil, a drug approved by the FDA for Narcolepsy, has begun to see widespread use in patients with MS. Unfortunately, the side effects of Provigil are similar to those of drinking 10 cups of cappuccino, and includes feeling ready to crawl out of your skin and start a hundred projects all at once. Think nervous little dog. Thankfully these side-effects lessen as a person gets used to taking Provigil.

The main way people with MS deal with their fatigue is moderation. This is accomplished by modifying your routine to times of day when you feel the most energized, breaking tasks down into small steps, and taking breaks when you feel tired. This is why I have only half my bills paid, while clean laundry sits in a basket on the floor, and I'm wearing one shoe. There are many articles out there, and in fact, whole chapters of books that discuss ways to live with your MS fatigue. This not one of them. Why? Because I'm too tired to think of any and I need to find my other shoe.

Instead, I am going to focus on discussing one of the other roadblocks in dealing with MS fatigue. Especially when it comes to getting medical care and understanding from those around us. The name. On the message board at MS MOMS, a common topic is how frustrating it is that our loved ones and doctors seem unable to comprehend the extent of our fatigue. I empathize completely. We are often called "lazy" or referred to as "whiners," by our own families because they chalk it up that we can't even deal with "a little bit of housework." This led me to the idea of a new name to combat the outsiders' perception of it.

First, when in discussion with any person who does not have MS, or any other disorder that causes chronic fatigue, the word fatigue itself is inadequate. When I looked up lethargic, a fancy word for tired, I got the word lazy as a synonym. This was a perfect example of how the rest of the world can link fatigue to laziness. I often find that when I mention fatigue to someone without MS, they tend to nod and say, "Uh-huh." While they are making the sounds of understanding, I can almost see a little bubble over their head saying, "Fatigued. No-one is ever that tired. She must be making excuses." Ignoring the fact that imagining bubbles appearing above people's heads is a bit nutty, you can see how difficult it can be to get friends and family to understand the severity of MS fatigue.

The lack of a good descriptive term for fatigue is also obvious in the medical world. Funny, because this is where I find understatement as common as wearing rubber gloves. My point:

73

"You will feel a little discomfort," when in fact I am probably going to experience searing pain and some sort of tool that looks like it should be in the tool shed not in a doctor's office. I thought that since doctors were used to doling out these understatements that surely they would know that when I say fatigue it does not mean "a little tired." However, the opposite seems to be true. I say fatigue and instead of thinking that I've been waylaid by the energy-sucking Monster, they think, "She's a little tired." I say this because it took me nearly a year to get my own neuro to prescribe fatigue medication and more than once I've heard fellow MSers upset because their doctor will not address their fatigue with something other than "Live with it."

The problem was clear. The word fatigue needed a face lift for those of us with MS. Then, we could all precisely explain to doctors and family what we're feeling. A fellow MS MOM once called it "profound exhaustion." I thought this term apt, but couldn't decide what was so profound about it unless, while lying on the floor, I considered the sudden insight that the patterns on the ceiling looked like clown faces. You don't even want to know what the swirls on the bathroom floor are doing.

Another woman made the typo of substituting the "G" for a "Q" so it read "fatique" pronounced fat-a-cue. This sounded very British and I imagined myself in one of those Edwardian A&E films sipping tea while saying, "It's not *fatigue*, mind you, it is fatique, which is much worse, I tell you." That was assuming I could round up the energy to make tea, which I can't. Since fatique, while sounding exotic, only ends up looking like a typo, my spell-checker is going nuts as we speak, I tossed the word away. In an attempt to come up with a better term, I looked up the word fatigue in a thesaurus and checked the synonyms. Nothing sounded like what I, and many others with Multiple Sclerosis, experienced.

My word needed to be intense. Every time I found a word, it

seemed lacking. Like my energy. I always came back to the words fatigue and exhaustion. But both sounded as if something outside myself had caused my state. They gave the impression of a life hangover; something I could simply "get over" if I took a long enough nap. Naps do help, but they do not make my fatigue magically go away.

Depleted, now that was a good word. So I settled on "depletion of strength." It conjured up images of dried out lakes, empty storage bins, and failed batteries. Yes, that was it! My batteries were not holding a charge. I was drained, or depleted, of energy. While angels did not sing a holy chorus when I decided on this phrase, I felt satisfied. My new way of explaining MS fatigue was with D.O.S. or Depletion of Strength.

After D.O.S. came my idea that to get my point across I could use something more than words. Maybe I could somehow show people how tired I felt. Investing in sallow green face paint might be a start. You know, the same stuff we slather on our faces at Halloween. If I made myself up to look like an extra from *Night of the Living Dead*, people just might get a clue. After all, I had the shuffling and moaning down, now I just needed the make-up to truly look like a zombie. This is called showing instead of telling. For those MSers willing to appear silly, it just might work!

Speaking of silly, one day my son was in the children's section of the bookstore. I joined him after finishing picking out my selection, and since he was sitting on the floor reading a book, so I sat on the floor with him. It also helped that I was currently experiencing extreme D.O.S. and the floor looked comfier than the tiny kid's chairs.

"Hey Mom, can I read this to you?" I looked over at the picture book he held and figured it would only take him a few minutes to read it.

"Go right ahead." Besides, Mark was not done with his shopping for a book on inner-peace, so I figured we had time. Stephan cheerfully began reading a book involving, if I recall correctly, a weasel and some other woodland creature. I stretched my legs in front of me and leaned back on my hands. His young voice ran on and on and I smiled at him, thinking of how comfortable the carpet was. Deciding that the children's section was made for lounging, I curled my knees up to my chest, wrapped my arms around them, and put my head down turned sideways so I could still see the pictures of the book. I convinced myself that I looked like a relaxed mother listening to her son read and didn't pay much attention to the other parents who were not on the floor. My son kept on reading and I closed my eyes to let his voice drift through my mind while I envisioned the story without the pictures. He paused.

"Mom? What are you doing?" When I peeked an eye open he was looking at me curiously.

"I'm just listening to you and letting the pictures show up in my head," I replied closing my eye again.

"But Mom the pictures are in the book!" I opened one eye again and smiled up at him.

"I know that, but I am making up my own pictures." I answered, stifling a yawn. He looked at me the way he does when I tell him sweeping is fun and then went back to reading. Once again I closed both eyes and listened to his voice.

"Mom." I sighed and did not open my eyes. After all I had already told him what I was doing. "Mom!" At his shout I relinquished and opened them.

"What?"

"I'm done," he said flatly. I yawned and rubbed my eyes. Darn

I had just been thinking about taking a nap.

"In fact, he finished that book and read a few others while you were peacefully snoring." Mark's voice cut into my thoughts. My head shot up from my knees and I looked around the bookstore shocked. Stephan had just started reading! What did he mean I was snoring?

As it turns out, Stephan had felt sorry for me and let me sleep. This is something I quickly learned about children. If you are at home and trying to nap they will find every reason under the sun to wake you up, but should you pass out in a public place they will go on about their business. There was a pile of books around him and Mark was sitting in one of those little kids chairs smiling down at me. I rubbed my eyes and glanced at my watch.

"How long was I out?"

"Four books, not including the one you fell asleep on," Stephan cheerfully replied.

"About 15 minutes," Mark added helpfully, getting up from his perch on one of those small chairs. I held up my hand and he helped me up off the floor. I could tell from the heat on my face that I was blushing like crazy. I wondered how many parents had walked by hearing me snore.

"Well then, now that I have proved the bookstore floor worthy of napping on, shall we go?" I attempted to look carefree when I felt like a complete fool. Mark laughed and patted me on the butt. Stephan asked if he could have "the book that puts Mom to sleep," and of course Mark told him yes. As we waited at the counter, I again yawned and leaned against Mark. The sales girl was looking at me with a huge grin and I wondered if while I was out, each employee had wandered past to look at the snoring lady. I quit returning her gaze and instead stared instead at my feet. Next to me, Mark laughed softly as if knowing what I was thinking.

When we got into the car I looked at him. "Did everyone hear me? I mean could you hear me across the store?"

"No, Babe. Not at all," he laughed.

"Was I really out that long?"

"Yep. A good ten or fifteen minutes."

"And you had your mouth open, too," Stephan offered from the back. I slunk down in my seat.

"Great. Snoring with my mouth wide open. The epitome of class and perfect parenting," I grumbled. How could I let myself fall asleep in a bookstore and on the floor no less! In one of their huge chairs I would have at least looked semi-normal.

"Well, you weren't snoring all that much. It was more like a soft growling," Mark offered in an attempt to console me. I wanted to die of embarrassment. I also felt like taking another nap.

"He's right, Mom. But only at first. Then it got louder and louder!" Stephan giggled. I shot a glare at Mark, who started laughing uproariously along with Stephan.

There is no miracle cure for D.O.S. Exercise and eating right can help in the area of willpower and stamina, also known as staying awake longer, but when the D.O.S. really kicks in, it could turn Jackie Joyner Kersey into a slug. So when someone looks at you like you're "just tired," I suggest, ignoring them, educating them on the facts of debilitating fatigue, or simply falling asleep on their shoulder and drooling.

Shhh... Bladder Problems

I think one of the most annoying and embarrassing symptoms I experience with Multiple Sclerosis is bladder trouble. While there are many avenues of medication and products to help with this situation, being 28 and having bladder problems is rather embarrassing. If anything I feel completely unattractive when I think about being a woman with bladder dysfunction. I have not resorted to catheters or sanitary undergarments yet, but I do foresee their presence in the future. For me, this is a completely depressing thought. People can't depend on me, but I'll be wearing Depends before I am 40.

If that wasn't bad enough, the exact trouble I have with my bladder, changes on a regular basis. The original problem, the urge to pee is always there. But how it comes out and how much, is an ever changing problem. Then my pee-pattern stepped up. I used to be able to do a 3-hour car ride with maybe one bath break. Now, I know every restroom and porta-potty from here to the northern coast of California. I've got a bathroom lined up for around every 30 minutes of the road trip.

I am also now the proud owner of various restroom anecdotes. I can remember the time I heard a toddler read aloud something inappropriate on a stall wall, but wouldn't you know I can't remember my appointments. I have also read things in stalls I wished I hadn't. There seems to be a promiscuous girl named Jenny who frequents all of my charted bathrooms. That also leads me to wonder why restrooms are called stalls. Of course, this phrase is very descriptive for me who can have problems where the pee stops partway, but for average people, why is the room we use to do our business named after a building where we store livestock? That seems simply wrong and unjust. Even a history lesson in bathrooms does not tell me why we went from "outhouse" to "stall". And I've tolerated some disgusting outhouses that make even the portable kind look pristine. I'm talking about a real old fashioned wooden shack in the middle of a field outhouse. Worse, I have peed beside my car in the middle of nowhere so often; I am beginning to wonder if I'm secretly an exhibitionist.

Speaking of stalls and exhibitionism let me get back to my problem. For those of you now thinking, "Oh, lord. Please, don't share!" you are free to move on to the next chapter. While this subject may be inappropriate and taboo, for many of us with MS it is a subject that needs to be addressed, because these things can and do happen in many of us. So here we go, into my bathroom and into the realms of too much information. Trust me; this is more painful for me than it is for you. You won't have to deal with your book being read and then having people say, "Look! There goes the pee lady."

Around year four a constant problem I dealt with was getting up in the middle of the night to pee. Or void. Or urinate. Whichever you feel is the best way to put it. No matter how you put it, it wasn't coming out. Sure, I woke up to rush to the toilet but then I would sit there with my insides freezing up, and me staring at the odd patterns on the tile floor. I knew that if I sat too long, my brain would go from hazy sleep mode into wide-awake mode so I would try thinking about water. If envisioning a rushing river did not help, I used the turn-on-the-sink trick. This became even trickier when trying to lean over and get the sink running without falling off the toilet.

I would wait, knowing I have to pee, because the urgency woke me out of a great dream involving ice cream and Sean Connery. Honestly, when your dreaming about getting cozy with a movie star, and then searching together endlessly for a usable bathroom, it's time to wake up and use the restroom.

This time, even the sink trick didn't work. By now, I'm convinced that if it takes much longer I am going to be wide awake at 4:00 a.m. This is when my brain decides to really click on. "Oh! She meant wake up!" So now, wide awake, I am practicing some relaxation techniques by moving my awareness inward and downward. My toes relax. My shins relax. My thighs relax. My stomach hangs over my knees, and suddenly it starts. A tingle. I get excited. It stops, and my butt cheeks go numb.

Most people would abandon this ordeal and head back to bed. But I know from previous experience that if I do, I will only be making the trek back to the bathroom within minutes. So I wait, sigh, and make a grocery list in my head. What drives me nuts is that these are the same muscles that at the movie theater seem incapable of holding one Dixie cup of fluid yet now are determined to show me they could hold back the entire contents of the Hoover Dam. I would be impressed if this was happening during daylight hours and a movie was showing. Instead, I find around this time that I am now doubting my sanity for having an inner argument with my body in the wee hours (pun intended) of the morning.

Finally, when I am back to making my grocery list, my muscles relax and the trial ends. I can pee, for five seconds. Then my body stops as if to say, "That was it. That's all we needed." I decide to wait a few more moments just in case. Like the rest of my indecisive nature, my body says, "Oh, wait! There's more!" But nothing happens, and I shuffle back to bed.

That done, more worries creep in because I am now awake. But before they do, there's that sensation of needing to use the bathroom again! This time, I ignore it by rolling over and wrapping myself around my body pillow. In this semi-fetal position, I let the concerns and random visions (There's that danged cat commercial again) float through my head until I drift back into fitful sleep.

Chapter 3

This was how things went for months. Sleeping pills helped me avoid a voiding spree in the middle of the night, but only kept it at bay until around 5:00 a.m. I attempted not to drink anything before bed. But this is difficult when you have five pills to take before bed. It didn't stop anyway. However, I really did not wish to go see my doctor. I didn't want to hear, "There's nothing wrong. It must be your MS," or "There is something wrong. It's your MS," or the grand finale, "Here. Have another pill."

I made do with what my body offered until, after three bladder infections, pain started. This pain, a burning sensation in the lower abdomen that passed quickly, had occurred a few times in the past. But now the pain was increasing and not going away. One day it was so intense that I stumbled, pants down to my bed and fell on to my stomach clutching myself. It felt like I had unwittingly fallen on a red-hot kabob. After about five minutes, the pain eased and Mark came into the room.

"Why are you flat on the bed with your pants down?" To him, I had only just been laughing and joking, moving about the house with a bustle of energy. When I explained through watery eyes what had happened. He puffed out his chest and took on the husband tone. "How long has this been going on?" I looked up at him and he moved to my feet to help me bring my pants back up.

"Well, it's never been this bad," I began.

"Never been this bad? You've had pain while urinating before?" This is where I got to puff up in response, because I had mentioned the pain before and obviously he did not remember. Typical man.

"I told you a few times that it hurt."

"You said it had something to do with your period and at this time, as far as I know, you're not on it! You are calling the doctor right now! I mean it!" He gave me the look he gives Stephan, our eldest, when he's in deep trouble. I sighed. He was right. But damned if I wanted to see the doctor. My new primary care doctor was a great man who understood MS. But while he knew that most often the only thing you can offer an MS patient is relief through medication, I still had not come to terms with it. But now, Mark realized what was going on and I had no choice. Sure, he noticed that I went to the bathroom often, but he had adjusted to this schedule, thinking there was nothing else to do. Pain was a different thing altogether. Pain, that had his wife doubled over on the bed, was not going to be ignored. So with Mark sitting in the same room looking at me sternly (which really only makes him look like Grizzly Adams), I called my primary.

At my visit, we discovered that I probably had a flaccid bladder. Flaccid was not a word I never thought could be associated with a woman in any way. Guess what? I left with a prescription. Apparently my bladder was not emptying all the way. Well, the many trips to the bathroom were a big tip off! Thoughts raced through my head and I attempted to keep my emotions under control as Mark drove us home. Once again, I had been almost symptom free. I had been working out and getting myself to a point where I actually had become what I always thought was a mythical creature, an MS jogger. The fatigue had backed off some, my feet were not tingling, my left eye was almost back to normal, my legs were working, and sure enough, the bladder thing started. Of course, it is a condition where the nerves are at fault. They are giving the bladder the wrong signals—just when I thought my MS was going to give me a break. Just when I had almost found "normal" again—I bit my lip to hold back tears. Who was I fooling? Normal was now something far from my reach.

After a few weeks on Detrol, with the pain still periodically occurring, the doctor did a test and found my bladder was still not emptying all the way. Let's just say this test involved a catheter and what looked like a small plastic bucket. Admitting that is humiliating enough, so I'm NOT going to drag you through the diagnosis blow by blow. This ended me with a referral to a PRD or Physical Rehabilitation Doctor. I liked to think of PRD as Pretty Rare Doctor, instead of a rehabilitation doctor. Especially after my primary described her as a person that works with people who have "spinal injuries, paraplegia, and people like you." What a way to bunch it all together and make me feel utterly broken, doc.

I went to see her. We dealt with a round of confusion as to why I was there for a bladder problem. She informed me that my flaccid bladder would not empty because I was having internal spasms. This was, of course, all due to my MS sending the wrong messages to my body. The solution? Here. Have another pill.

Before I could scream, whine, and stomp my feet, she told me this new miracle pill guaranteed to help my quality of life was Baclofen. Wait a minute, I knew that name. It was a muscle relaxant that I had listed in my articles and web site as the pill to deal with spasticity in MS. When I thought "spasm," I had always thought of my leg shooting out from under me and doing the jitterbug, not inner parts. According to the PRD, inner parts could spasm just as well as outer parts. Oh, goody! Yet another invisible symptom! She also comforted me with the knowledge that she had other MS patients on the same pill for this exact problem. I think the only reason I'd never heard about it in this context was because no one was daft enough to bring it up in conversation. Or in writing. Until now.

As I walked back out with yet another prescription, I tried to look on the bright side of things. This is a very hard thing to do when you're talking about bladder problems, catheters, and spasticity. I tired to think of no more catheter tests, no surgery, and no more pain. Mark, noting my serious face, nudged me.

I glanced over and he put his arm around my shoulders. In his best Homer Simpson voice he said "Mmmmm! Muscle Relaxants! Ooohhh." Our laughter was my bright side.

Optic Neuritis

One day my eye began to twitch. Everyone gets eye-twitches. Usually, I am sure my eye is flapping around in its socket, yet everyone else says "what eye twitch?" You know that eye twitch. Did I mention the word twitch? However, this time my eye did not cease its convulsing after the requisite amount of time, but instead kept going. Having an eye spasm that is completely unrecognizable to those around you is simply annoying. It makes you doubt your sanity. So, I stood in the bathroom staring at my eye until I finally caught a slight quiver. Then I was able to yell "HA! You see? It IS moving!" I forced my husband, Mark, to stare at my face until, he too, confessed that there was a tiny shudder in my eyeball. "Houston we have socket movement", and I am not insane.

Twitch confirmed, I called my neurologist sure that this was a sign that my optic nerve was falling apart. You never know when those little white cells have taken up residence in your nerves for the all-you-can eat myelin buffet. Of course, like every other symptom, when it came time to see the doctor, the eye quit moving. Why does that always happen? Is it some kind of white cell stage fright?

Needless to say, my neuro was not impressed. "Eye twitches are a normal muscular function often times worsened by stress. By the way, not everything that goes wrong with your body is caused by MS." Darn it! I was just about to blame my PMS on MS. P is easily added. Hey why not a new definition for MSers "P-MS"- it's Probably MS!

This advice made me feel a bit like a hypochondriac. So I swore to myself that someday soon, I would return triumphant. My eye would leap from its socket, and I would walk into the doctor's sterile office, with my dangling eyeball and say, "Now tell me THIS is normal!" In the meantime, I spent my days stopping time whenever my eye convulsed. This made for awkward shopping cart moments in the grocery store.

To my dismay, my eyeball did not leap from its encasement and the shuddering did stop. I was forced to consider the possibility that I was being a tad hyper-vigilant, and needed to admit that, just possibly, not everything that went wrong with my body was the fault of my multiple sclerosis. I begrudged the thought that everyone who had uttered the words "that happens to everyone" or "simply accept that you have MS and move on" could have a point. Was I simply a hypochondriacal basket case?

A month or so later, I began to experience sharp shooting pains in my left eye whenever I moved it or touched it. Since it was in the same eye that had spent a month doing the jitterbug, I vowed that I would not blame it on MS. Instead, I went to my allergist.

I proclaimed that the pain was caused by what I felt was another sinus infection. Being allergic to dogs and cats, yet unable to part with my pets, it was quite a regular occurrence for me to be stuffed up and experiencing sinus pain. The allergist looked me over and proclaimed that I did not have a sinus infection, but my nose was a "+4", and my tongue had "cobblestoning". [And I thought my neurologist came up with some odd medical descriptions.) He gave me a prescription for antibiotics under the strict promise that I would only fill it if my symptoms got worse.

After arriving home, I determined that saying my nose was +4 was not a sly medical term for saying I had a large honker. I considered the possibility that something even simpler was causing the pain. Too much time at the computer? Nevertheless, I had to turn my head to look at things because even small movement of the eye was painful. Within a few days, things got better -and worse- all at the same time.

At first when I woke up, I thought my eye was filled with sleep, so I kept rubbing it, to clear it up. The pain had backed off a little, so I figured that I was on the way to recovery from whatever problem had caused the pain. But what the heck was with the odd feeling that there was some sort of film over my left eye? I sent my son off to school and went to the gym with my husband, all the while rubbing my eye.

It was when I was clutching the treadmill for dear life that I noticed it was difficult to read a sign attached to the TV in front of me. Time for a test. I closed my left eye and looked out of my right. Clear and crisp letters on the sign. Slowly I closed my right and opened my left. Blurry. I let go with one hand and rubbed at my eye, causing me to lean in the opposite direction and quickly drop my hand to steady myself before I slid off the back of the treadmill. Like a kid who has suddenly realized that you can see different views from each eye; I began to switch back and forth between the views.

Yep. The left eye was blurred. After my workout, the blurring seemed to increase. I debated mentioning it to Mark because he would most likely tell me to call my neuro and I did not want to be told it was some normal phenomena due to stress. Besides, the pain had backed off tremendously, so where was the harm in a little blurring? Maybe I had simply burnt out my eye bulb with computers, reading and sitting too close to the TV. After all, everyone in my family wore glasses, well except my sister, and my brother and— it didn't matter! I was not going to be an MS hypochondriac. I resolved that I needed glasses and would make an appointment with the optometrist.

On the way home however, I could not resist closing one eye

and then the other. Considering that I often do oddball things, it took Mark a bit to notice my antics, but he did. In the middle of making a turn, he glanced over at me.

"What are you doing?"

"Hmm? Nothing. Just looking out one eye and then the other. It's kind of fun." I glanced at him and he gave me a suspicious look.

"How's your eye today? Still hurting?"

"Not so much." I noticed my voice went up an octave this usually belies my nervousness. Mark's eyes were not blurry.

"So what's bugging you?"

"Why would think that anything is bugging me? Look at the road."

"Oh, I don't know. Maybe it's because you started this morning by rubbing at your eye like you had some sort of tic and since you were on the treadmill you've been looking out one eye and then the next as if your comparing." I had the grace to look sheepish.

"You saw that?" I asked amazed again that my husband notices these small changes. He nodded. I puffed. "The pain has backed off. It's now sort of dull instead of sharp, but my vision in that eye is blurry. It's like there is a film over my eye. Even colors seem off."

"You need to call Dr. S," he stated.

"No. I don't. I do not need him telling me it is nothing. It's probably sinuses putting pressure on my eye ball or something." I didn't even convince myself with that story.

"All right. When we get home you look in the green hypo-chondriac book and if it says nothing about MS and every-thing about sinus trouble, I'll believe you."

I grimaced and nodded.

The green hypochondriac book was a heavy tome of the world's worst diagnoses. It listed symptoms and then every possible disease, thus its name: the hypochondriac book. A person could look up sore finger in that green monster of a book and instead of reading about splinters, they could diag-nosis themselves with carpal tunnel or even gangrene. Okay Mark and I are macabre, nay pessimistic at times, so we keep the thing around. We like to call it realism.

The heavy book balanced on my lap, I flipped through until I got to eye pain. First choice: with discharge or "copious tear-ing." I had neither. I moved on to "without eye discharge or copious tearing." Wait! What exactly did copious mean? Could it mean filmy? I consulted a dictionary just to waste time. But soon enough found my list of potential diseases.

My first choice was Chlamydia, an infectious disease cause by a group if microorganisms called Chlamydia. Otherwise known as an STD, or sexually transmitted disease. How in the heck does a person get that in their eye? All manner of horrible visions had to be banished from my head as I scrolled down the list. Eye cancer, glaucoma, migraine, optic neuritis. Oh crap. Optic Neuritis.

I'd read that term before. Wasn't that the way most people with MS were diagnosed? I recalled that in the first few years, my neuro kept asking after my vision. To my credit, sinusitis was listed directly underneath the dread OP. I read both de-scriptions and knew I had lost my bet with Mark. If I had been experiencing sinusitis, my allergist would have diagnosed it. Optic neuritis read exactly like what I had been experiencing:

blurred vision, pain in the affected eye.

When I flipped to the back of the green monster where the lengthier descriptions of each disease resided, I frowned as I read the symptoms of OP: impaired color perception in one or both eyes. Pain when moving or touching affected eye, especially within the first few days of symptoms. Partial or total vision loss. The next sentence sealed my call to the neuro. "An episode of optic neuritis may be one of the earliest indications of multiple sclerosis." I'd had MS for around 4 years at this point. Gee, I thought, "everyone in my family might not need glasses but we are habitually late."

Within a few days, I was once again in the neurologist's office, sitting in the chair that the patient is required to sit in, while Mark got the comfy couch. Bright light shone in my eye as my neurologist got closer to my face than he'd ever been before. He mentioned that the nerve did not appear swollen and I wondered how he could even see it. Next a brief eye exam. I read from a card with one eye and then the other. The blurring was definitely altering my ability to see through the eye. Next was a color test in wherein I confirmed that colors were darker with my left eye.

After writing a prescription for steroids, the neurologist leaned back in his seat perturbed. He scolded me, "Why didn't you come in when the pain started?" I looked at Mark. He rolled his eyes and I said "You know, Doctor, not everything that goes wrong with my body is caused by MS." Mark and I knew it was just P-MS. (Probably MS.)

Confessions of an MS Jogger

Since my diagnosis, I often run into people who cheerfully tell me about "their friend with MS, who jogs." I take this to mean that I am not allowed to be waylaid by my MS, or to have any cumbersome symptoms. Like the MS jogger, I am to defeat MS with exercise and good life choices. This phrase, "good life choices" always, and I mean ALWAYS makes me crave doughnuts or pizza. My school psychologist used to recommend "good life choices," and back then it always made me crave a cigarette. Those well-meaning people who tell me about their never-been-stopped-by-a-little-MS friends figure that if their friend is unaffected, then I shouldn't have problems either. After all, MS effects everyone the same way, right?

Either that or the whole thing is really the "buck up" speech. You know that speech. It's the one from the movies. The one where an actor is lying on a snowy mountain with a broken leg and the other actor is telling him, "You've got to keep moving! Don't let this defeat you! We can still make it out of here." Considering my distant relation to the Donner party, and my aforementioned inability to make good life choices, my reaction to the buck up speech is to eat the well-intentioned friend and wait comfortably for rescue.

That is about how much faith I had in the idea that I'd ever do any sort of vigorous exercise again. Forget the off chance that my legs would occasionally hold up under an attempt to move faster than a brisk walk. I didn't think I'd ever have enough energy to jog again. I knew that people who do aerobics with MS existed, but I assumed their MS was just not as bad as mine was. MS-exercisers seemed unrealistic to me, just like the models in ads for MS pharmaceuticals: thin, good-looking and always out hiking or on bikes. These ads make statements that encourage sufferers to "take back" their life or to make "their own future." Wonderful concept. But it requires that the patient, for instance me, actually feel that a chance actually existed to get life back.

After three years, the idea that I might someday be where I was in 1999, jogging, driving, running a household, and working traveling sales in my husband's Renaissance Faire business was laughable. To even utter an idea like "I am going to eat right, exercise, and my MS will simply go away" smacked of denial and would only have served to alarm my husband and give my counselor another reason to tack on five more sessions. I am still not sure how talking about my mother for 30 days helps me to cope with my condition, but that's another essay. So, I settled for a life that was less than and a body that was less than. To me, it was no biggie.

At least, not at first. During my first diagnosed year, I was so wrapped up in being sure that I was going to die that I didn't have time to consider exercising. Unless I was bemoaning the loss of my ability to exercise. The last thing I wanted to do in my fatigue was exercise. Besides, it wouldn't complement my chosen coping mechanism: eating. Screw eating sensibly, my body was messed up anyhow! I'd take a pizza with everything on it and a pitcher of beer with my friends. I decided to battle my disease with humor AND chocolate. Besides, it's a softer landing to fall onto a couch than a treadmill if your legs quit on you!

For three years my idea of exercise was yelling (neck muscles) into the next room and shopping trips for 30 minutes at a pace of 0.5. I did diet when I could not fit into my fat clothes. But those diets consisted of going back to smoking cigarettes and drinking coffee instead of eating. Overall, my love of junk food and my refusal to link mind and body kept me in extra padding, just in case I fell.

I embraced my job as family photo taker because then the pictures would not show my double chin or double butt. I watched myself go from a young woman, always posing for the camera, to a woman whom, if caught and forced into a photo, held up her head to diminish her double chin. It was sad. Sad enough to make me eat another pint of ice cream.

Then came December 2002 and my niece's birthday party. I always enjoyed visiting my eldest brother and his wife. Not just because they are family, but also because they were big and comfortable. They loved food and disliked exercise as much as I did. Plus, they had two children. I have recently discovered that two children, no matter their ages, cause an undeniable urge to eat and sleep.

But at that party, I came face to face with a much thinner brother and sister-in-law. I could have wept. They both looked to have dropped around 20 pounds I wanted to tell them this was mutiny! But Mark, too, had begun to complain about his weight the way men do, by walking around with a knit sweater covering only half his belly and looking like a cartoon character. I grudgingly asked how they did it and how much time I would have to spend wheezing in the great outdoors. They said they never exercised. I said sign me up.

Somewhere between following a new diet that involved no exercising and my favorite foods, beef and cheese, Mark and I started to take walks. This was much to the enjoyment of our dog, who had begun to jump the fence and walk himself. Hand in hand, we would slowly make our way around the cement pathway of the local park. The dog still felt betrayed, though, because we walked so s-l-o-w.

Eventually, partially motivated by boredom and imploring looks from our dog, we ventured to the part of the park with dirt paths and many trees. In the early morning hours, while Stephan was at school we would walk in the woods around the park and let the dog have his fun. Usually, while I looked down at my feet making sure I did not trip on anything, or get hung up on low branches, we would spend the time discussing trivial things like how the dog acted. One day, though, we began to discuss money.

Somewhere at the top of the list of ten reasons couples fight is money. We must have somehow thought we were impervious to these statistics, because there we were, ambling down a dirt path in the middle of winter talking about how to lessen our bills. It all began innocently enough, but in a rather snippy tone Mark suddenly said, "Well if we didn't spend so much on fast food we might actually be able to save."

To me, them was fightin' words. It was a clear accusation that my addiction to eating was the reason we didn't own a house, or a brand new car, and why we were so out of shape in the first place. "It is not as if I twist your arm to make you drive to MacDonald's," I shot back, pushing up the sleeves to my sweatshirt as if getting ready for a fist fight. From where he walked behind me, as he customarily did, Mark went silent.

He said he walked behind me in case I fell. That seemed odd, because I knew that falling usually involved my lurching for-ward not backward. Why I suddenly thought about this, and how I decided it meant that he thought I was fat because he didn't want me falling on him at that exact moment is one of those things I like to call: being female. Now I was not only wasting the family's money and force feeding him MacDonald's, but I was unattractive. Fat equals unattractive, right?

"You are right, I could say no. But if I say no, you get mad and it's easier to get the food." He remarked quickening his step to catch up with me as I began to pick up our usual strolling pace.

"Oh! So the whole reason we're fat is because I MAKE you eat fast food!" I growled, my feet moving just a bit quicker with the adrenaline now beginning to course through my body. I thought about how unfair he was being and how hideous he thought I was. No wonder he spurned my advances the other morning as we lay in bed. Sure he said he had migraine, but that's what women say

"I thought we were talking about saving money." Mark called from behind me. "I never said you were the reason we're fat." That was it.

"So you do think I'm fat!" I exclaimed, loud enough to make our dog pause and check if I was hollering at him for some reason.

"Well, we both admitted to gaining weight. I know you haven't felt very attractive recently."

"Hah! I knew you found me unattractive!" Although I had already assumed he found my looks to be lacking, it hurt more to hear what I thought was him confirming it. Suddenly I wanted nothing more than to get away from Mark. It was either that, or locate an item to lob at his head. Never mind the a little voice inside my head that was screaming something about jumping to conclusions and being unreasonable.

"What?" He sounded stunned. But it was fleeting. After all, this man had been with me for eight years. "That's not what I said!" Mark replied, his voice also rising. "I said you thought you were unattractive. And you know better!" He paused to call the dog back from an attempt to wander too close to the road, and then continued after me. "How did we get from saving money to me thinking you were fat and unattractive?" Again he paused as if mulling the question over in his head. I continued walking no longer paying attention to the path but instead consumed by the argument. "Are you PMS-ing?"

"Of course!" I stopped walking and turned to look at him. He was a few feet behind and his cheeks were red. "If I say anything that you don't understand, I have to be PMS-ing or insane, or just having cognitive difficulties!"

"Well you do have cognitive difficulties-",

"That's not my point!" I shrieked.

"Exactly! And my point was that we could eat less out. I never said anything about you being unattractive. So tell me how you got from saving money to being the ugly and fat." Mark gave me that proud look that signals he feels he has proven me to be unreasonable. This meant I had to show exactly how I got to my point.

"You walk behind me." I muttered.

"I- what?" Now he looked off kilter, which meant I had the upper-hand.

"Yes. You walk behind me-"

"In case you fall!"

"Since when do women trip on things in front of them and fall backward?" I replied calmly, noting that for some reason I felt a tad out of breath.

"It keeps you from knocking me down-" A dawning look of realization came across Mark's face. "So, you think you're fat." I nodded and crossed my arms across my chest. He stifled a grin. "It is possible for me to see you falling and catch you in time," he continued.

When Mark saw the "yeah right" look on my face he quickly continued, "I mainly walk behind you to watch how you are walking. I can then tell if you are swerving, limping, all of that. It lets me know how well you are doing." Mark then placed an arm about my waist. A risky move, considering I had been ready to throw something at him. "Besides the view is better," he remarked patting my behind. I tried not to grin. "Do you know", he asked as he turned me in the direction of the parking lot "that you just walked at a rather quick pace and never even stumbled?"

"I did?" I replayed the tiny argument in my mind. I had taken off and continued at a brisk pace, without falling. The parking lot at the other end of the park was now further away because of how far I had marched off into the woods. "I wonder how that happened."

"We've been exercising and you've been eating right. I think your mind works better the healthier you are, maybe it even works better at repairing itself. I think we should join a gym and really see what you can do." I paused in our trek to the car and looked at him as if he'd grown another head.

"Seriously. They'd have a swimming pool which would not put strain on your muscles, and you can hold on to the handlebars of treadmills. Plus they would have a trainer who would know what sort of low intensity weight lifting you could do to help tone you up." I elbowed him in the stomach and he laughed. "Me too! I need toning too."

"What about saving money? Weren't you just complaining that we wasted money on fast food?"

"If we take the money we would eat in fast food and put it away, maybe I can afford a gym membership for us." He gave me a teasing look, "but you have to promise to stop force-feeding me burgers."

"Only if you quit shoving chow mien down my throat."

The gym was designed for families, but all I saw on the day Mark and I wandered in, was thin women in tight outfits. Mark looked around taking everything in, and I shook my head.

"I can't do this. Look at her. Is that a thong?" I have finally conceded that women wear thong underwear despite its purpose to ride up their butt. To me that has always been an unpleasant experience and something you cannot remedy in public places. However, wearing a thong leotard was just too close to wearing underwear on the outside: something that either required the body of a Victoria's Secret model, or just plain insanity. Mark noted the direction of my eyes and nudged me. He leaned over and pointed at some men who looked like extras from a Conan movie, oiled biceps, and all.

"And I look like them?" he laughed. "Come on it will be fine. This place is for families and we haven't seen the whole gym yet."

Our guide, a toned young man who could barely be 20 (let's call him Chad) led us upstairs while prattling on about the rock climbing wall. I understand that the gym wanted its representatives to look fit and that this would encourage possible members to join, but when you feel that the rep is a "kid," it can be hard to feel comfortable. It's worse when not only is the rep a kid, but the he and the rest of the people meandering about look like living breathing Ken and Barbie dolls. I wanted to turn tail and walk, not run, because that would involve stairs and coordination, walk back to my house and eat.

When we crested the top of the stairs I noticed an immediate difference. Amongst the Barbies, there were women of other shapes and ages. The men varied as well. Along the two rows of treadmills some ran and some walked while clinging to the handle bars. That would be me, I thought as I watched a woman who looked about 80. Chad caught my look and pointed to a room off to the side where only women were allowed to enter.

I wondered if this bothered the men, not having their own place to hide out and exercise, but later discovered that basically the whole lower floor was always dominated by men, with oily biceps.

We were seated inside a tiny room with the door open. This helped me continue to let my ADD-like attention wander away from the conversation that had too many technicalities anyhow. The possibility that I might actually be able to handle walking on a treadmill and lifting weights was tantalizing. Before my diagnosis in 1999, I had been working out on a regular basis for a year. Of course, I never realized how well I was looking until later when I saw photos. Excitement ran through me as I imagined slipping into my favorite jeans without any gasping or the use of hand-held tools. Coat hanger through zipper? It was an 80s thing.

My ears tuned back into the conversation when Chad began asking questions about our current eating habits and exercise level. I pondered asking if he'd seen what bears do before hibernation and snorted at my own imaginings while Mark nudged me under the table. He knew that any sort of snort or snicker usually meant my answer was not for public hearing. Next, were the questions about health problems. I highly doubted our handsome Chad had a clue what MS was, but I decide to go with being nonjudgmental and hoping that they had covered MS somewhere in their training. What is their training anyway? Do you have to drop and do 100 push-ups? Is it like boot-camp?

"My wife has Multiple Sclerosis," Mark replied.

"So you'd like a membership for her as well?" Chad jotted down a note. Mark looked at me, and I shrugged.

"Well of course," he said.

"All of our facilities are wheelchair accessible," Chad added.

"Well she's hardly in a wheel-" Mark began, but Chad looked up at me and smiled.

"So then you'd like a membership for your daughter as well?" Mark looked confused.

"Angie?" Mark looked at me for help. I had a feeling I knew where Chad was going wrong. Mark and I have a 14 year age difference, but I kept it to myself. Chad grinned at me again.

"Angie? That is a beautiful name you have." I laughed loudly and Mark finally caught on.

"She's not my daughter! She's my wife!" Mark snorted, from somewhere between laughing and being insulted. Chad looked dismayed.

"But. She has Multiple Sclerosis?" Mark and I nodded. "Isn't Multiple Sclerosis where you can't walk and have a short time to live?"

"No." I responded, with a straight face. "Only my victims have that problem." Mark elbowed me and I rolled my eyes. Chad looked even more confused. He then asked if my condition would interfere with regular exercise. I muttered something about getting to the fridge just fine, while Mark gave the actual answer. He rattled off that I could not get overheated, that I needed low intensity weights, if any, and that I should not put tons of stress on my body. Chad looked at me and as if to make up for his lack of education about MS and said "Well you look pretty good."

Mark suddenly had possession of both my hands under the table in a grip strong enough that I would not be able to lunge for young Chad's throat. The "looking good" comment had been the bane of my existence since I was diagnosed. I looked too good to be ill, too good to be fatigued, and definitely too good to be disabled.

The whole situation was surreal. I was too out of shape and too MS-y to be in a gym. Just because I walked fast while I was angry didn't mean I could keep it up. Just because I had felt pretty good for the last month did not mean I wouldn't be back in the hospital next month. This was presumptuous. I was acting as if I could simply jog and get on with life. And I wasn't ready to let go of my original coping mechanism: eating.

A week later, after many booster speeches from Mark, I got the courage up to go to the gym. Feeling like a very pitiful woman in my sweats and long t-shirt, I followed Mark up the stairs to the average-looking-people workout room. By the time we topped the two flights of stairs, my calves were sore. I asked if we could be done and use going back down the stairs as our cool down. Mark reminded me that I had walked further on our strolls and I informed him that there was a big difference between "strolling" and "exercising."

Mark ignored my grumbling and picked two side by side treadmills in a line of 5. I tried to look nonchalant and in charge as I stepped on and began pushing buttons. One would think that a treadmill is an easy piece of equipment to operate, but this is not always true. Chad had shown us how to start the type of treadmill I was on, and so I had pushed what I thought was the correct button to enter my age and weight. The machine lurched to life and the belt began moving.

"Ack!" I gripped the handrails in front of me and looked to Mark for help.

"Don't look so panicked. You're walking at a slower speed than you normally do," he commented, already walking at a brisk pace on his machine. The people on the other 3 machines were now glancing over at me because of the yelp I had let out. Great. Now everyone knew I was a novice! The heart rate monitor that was also the handle bars I had a death-grip on, showed a spike in my beat. I wondered if I could get myself into an aerobic heart rate by just panicking, that way I could do it at home without people staring at me.

"How do I make it go a wee bit faster?" I asked, trying to focus on walking, gripping and Mark all at the same time. Mark nodded at the buttons. I pushed the speed button and nothing seemed to happen. So with one hand holding on and the other manning the buttons, I decided I needed to hold my finger down on the pad in order to raise speed. I succeeded. The machine went from .5 to 2.5 in an instant.

At least this time I didn't scream. Instead I held on for dear life and tried to look as if I meant to cause such a big jump in speed. A speed of 2.5 is not all that fast, mind you, but I didn't feel in control on the treadmill. In the park I could look at my feet, watch for bumps in the path, and control my speed. On a treadmill, looking at my feet as the belt moved could make me motion sick. Also, there were all these buttons to be pushed with the one hand that wasn't holding on as if gale force winds had blown through the room. This particular machine's heart monitor yelled at you by way of big letters to put your hands back down if you lifted them, too! I never thought a machine could give me a guilt complex!

However, I was determined to master this beast and not continue looking like an idiot. Of course, I was the only person on the top floor who felt that everyone was watching and determining that I was an idiot and handicapped, to boot. It occurred to me that this may have been the first time in history that a room full of people decided I truly was physically challenged. While attempting to get my feet into a rhythm with the machine, preferably one that did not include falling, I tried to

103

discover what I should be looking at.

I knew from earlier inspection, before I was trapped on a machine with a moving floor, that people were either listening to headphones or watching the TV that hung from the ceiling. To look at the TV, though, I had to tilt my head up and back. I knew this would result in either a sore neck or a sore bottom. I already knew from previous collisions at the grocery store that looking to the left or right while moving usually resulted in my swerving that direction. Eventually I decided to keep my eyes locked where they were, straight ahead. Across the room past the weight machines, was a wall paneled with mirrors. I focused on a chubby woman with a green bandana who looked ready to faint, until I realized it was my reflection. While wondering if the mirrors were there as a sort of cruel incentive to keep moving, I turned my eyes downward to the machines control panel. How does this thing work, anyway?

Apparently, my original problem had started by hitting the "quick start" button. I noticed Mark moving out of the corner of my eye. He had gotten off his machine and was now leaning over mine. Had it already been ten minutes?

"Are you going to turn it down?" he asked casually. I gave him a quick glance and saw he was grinning. I dearly wished I had a free hand.

"Why would I turn it down?" I asked with a snooty tone.

"Maybe because it is going too fast for you?"

"It is not going too fast. I set it at this speed." I remarked, noticing that I did not sound as calm as I wished. I had begun to breathe harder to keep up the pace. Surely people were watching now. I had a man leaning on my treadmill.

"So that's why you're panting and your knuckles have turned

white?" Mark reached for the panel and pushed the button to slow my speed.

"Hey! Get your hands off my machine!" I called out, forgetting my fear and swatting lightly at his hand. Now people were looking. My walking slowed with the machine and I tossed a semi-glare at Mark as he slowly brought the treadmill to a stop. He smiled and winked at me, knowing that I was not truly angry. He also knew what was coming next.

A funny thing about the brain and treadmills. When the treadmill stops moving, the brain says you're still going. Kind of like the feeling you get when you're in the car wash. The car isn't moving the brushes are, but your brain will tell you the car is in motion. When a person attempts to walk normally after being on a treadmill, they do one of two things: exit gracefully, or walk as if they've had a few drinks. I'm betting you can guess what I did. When I stepped off the machine and tried to take a step forward, I tilted.

Mark put his hands on my arms to steady me just as a gym employee approached us. I was sure someone had noted the woman struggling on the treadmill and called for help. I was surprised that it was only one employee that had come to drag me off the machine and not a squad of paramedics. I gave a weak smile to the burly man and waited for him to give me a lecture on safe treadmill practices. Instead, he pulled Mark aside. I was getting rather irritated at being treated like an infant thinking that the employee should be talking to me and not my husband about my sad display on the equipment, when Mark came back to my side.

"Apparently it is against gym policy to pick up women. I've been ordered to quit harassing you."

I would have died laughing, if I wasn't already out of breath.

Months later after the security incident at our gym, I was walking on the treadmill like a pro. I was now in good enough shape to walk for 20 minutes at a very quick pace. The speed that had me panting in the beginning, 2.5, was now closer to a warm-up speed. Because the program was regulated by my heartbeat and the goal was to keep me at an aerobic pace, it became necessary to raise the incline of the machine as I walked. I often told Mark that this was the only time a person could say they had to walk a mile that was uphill both ways. It was either walk at an incline or jog, and no matter how comfortable I was now with fast-walking on the treadmill –while still holding on the whole time-I was not going to attempt jogging and tripping in front of a room full of people.

Mark and I were in pretty good shape. We both benefited from diet and exercise. I hated to admit it, as much as I loved hot fudge sundaes, but eating right and exercising seemed to help my MS as well. Despite a bout of optic neuritis in the winter, my symptoms had basically remitted. My fatigue was still present but it didn't kick in until the afternoon. From 8:00 am to around 2:00 pm each day, I felt close to normal.

We continued our walks in the park and as spring arrived, we often picked the outdoors over the gym. One day, as we puffed our way down the path, Mark commented that I was going to have to quit using the treadmills at the gym. When I asked why, he remarked that if I put my incline any steeper I would be walking at a 90 degree angle.

"If I don't set the incline high, I don't get my heart rate up enough."

"Increase the speed." Mark responded, also increasing his pace. He was now jogging at a slow pace.

"I can't!" I called, chasing after him.

"Why not?" He called back over his shoulder.

"Because then I would be jogging." I caught up to him and pumped my arms to keep my pace along side his. He smiled at me.

"And to think months ago you could barely walk down this path! Now you can almost keep up with me." Mark gave me a challenging grin. "Of course, you'll never be faster than me." He turned and loped down the path. I tried to walk even faster but found my legs were going as fast as they could. So I added a spring to my step and loped a few feet myself. When my legs didn't collapse beneath me and Mark yelled back another challenge. "You're the tortoise. I'm the hare!"

Now I won't say that it was simple or that I was graceful. I wobbled and weaved and generally felt like I was trying to move someone else's body, but I was damned if I was going to let Mark disappear over the horizon that easy. When I rounded the bend I saw him heading toward a stone bench. He called out that his was the finish line. As I continued moving at a steady pace, watching Mark get closer to the finish, it dawned on me that I had been wasting my time. Even though I was attempting something like a jog, I was holding back. I was playing it safe, just in case my body tricked me.

I had been playing it safe for three years, always aware that my body could trick me at any moment and take away any progress I had regained. After taking a few spills in my first year, I had learned to fear. Not only had I become overly cautious when I was fatigued, but I didn't trust my body even when I was feeling good! I regarded my own limbs with mistrust and suspicion. I never completely let loose because I "might" fall. I had learned to think that if I had fallen once, I would always fall. But that day, something shifted. For a few moments in time, I didn't care if I fell. I simply wanted to win. I wanted to BE the elusive MS Jogger. I wanted to be the spokes model for the pharmaceuticals. So I let go and hauled ass.

I didn't beat him by any means, and I felt like my heart was going to come out my nose as I lay down on the bench. I rested my head in Mark's lap, but for that moment, there was no disability. There was no fear. Just an imaginary finish line that had taken 3 years to cross. As I stared up at the oak trees, I began to wonder if this was how MS joggers did it. I always assumed that the people with MS who jogged were completely free of symptoms. It never occurred to me that they may have the same kind of MS, except when they were doing well they didn't hole up at home in fear of the next bad day. Instead, maybe they went jogging. From that day on no matter how many times I ended up on my butt, I did not live in fear of my own body.

Depression

For those of you, who wanted to gag while reading about my blissful reconnection with exercise, be consoled. Within a month, I was back in my bedroom, swaddled with my favorite blanket and watching chick flicks while stuffing my face. Falling off the health wagon is very easy when you have the willpower of a puppy. Have you ever left a package of meat on the table and expected Fido NOT to steal it? Willpower aside, launching off the wagon as if being bit in the butt and landing face down in a pint of ice cream is even easier when depressed. Because despite what theatrical musicals will tell you, a little whistle and a dance routine do not make your troubles go away. Instead, you just break your ankle when you try to do that little move of clicking your heels together.

Within a month, I was back on my butt and not eager to hop back up again. I don't remember exactly what rekindled my love for the couch, an illness, or an argument, but it had been enough. Of course, with my willpower, one toe stubbed while collecting a mailbox full of bills, can send me right to the phone for pizza delivery and then straight to the bed for some quality time with my remote. One moment I've hit my stride and am getting pretty darn proud of how well I am learning to live with my condition, and the next I'm contemplating the red sauce stain on my sheets. The best way to beat back the tired feeling at the end of a bad day is to make it all better with a binge night in my bedroom.

My usual binge consists of going to the video store renting enough movies to qualify me for the deal with candy, popcorn, and a giant soda. Then head to the grocery store to load up on the main course. Popcorn and candy are just appetizers. You may think that only chocolate can induce a peaceful feeling but large amounts of carbohydrates in the form of pizza, chips, and sizable amounts of spicy Cheezits, can also make a person feel giddy. It's either the chemicals in the food or the sudden lack of caring about diet that creates this bliss. Therefore my menu can range from a hot fudge sundae to chips and salsa, with a margarita of course.

It never occurred to me while I was shopping for my chewable uppers that the bag of chips or box of ice cream would still be in the house the next day to tempt me. I simply thought "I'm in good shape. I deserve this after a bad day." Or "I'll work it off later." I always thought that people who were in top shape worked out because they loved it. Now I know that most of us constantly have to force ourselves to go out. Once I get going I feel better, but getting my rear in gear is hard. This makes it like work. Thus the words working out are very appropriate. The way I usually see it, if it's like work, it's not worth it. They say anything worth having is worth working for. I say if you can get it while lying on the couch, much better. But I digress.

This time around I was rapidly sliding off the health wagon while happily snacking on chips. After binging I tried to go back to my regular routine until another thing set me off. After a period of weeks, symptoms began to pop up that led to more time down. Symptoms up, body down, pounds on. I should have known what was coming next. Depression.

After about a steady week of hanging out in my bedroom flipping absently through the 875 channels on my TV because we always need 874 channels with nothing on, Mark brought up the subject one afternoon.

"Do you think you might be depressed?" I glanced up from a fascinating commercial about a grandmother with rock hard abs and frowned at him.
"Nope."

"You've been in bed for a week babe."

"Have not."

"Oh really? What have you been doing then?"

"Resting in-between bathroom trips." I gave him a sassy grin. His frown deepened. There is nothing more pleasing to a depressed person than dragging someone down with them. That and picking on other happy, well-adjusted people.

"Love, you've been binge eating, you've quit working out, and to be honest you're a crabby bi-," he paused and made a helpless motion with his hands that I took for charades.

"Sounds like itch?" I asked, craning my neck to see around him and whether or not Jerry Springer had come back on. Nothing better than watching people worse off than you.

"You need to do something." He remarked turning off the TV before coming by the bed.

"Oh, that was cruel. I was just about to find out if the baby was the neighbor's or the husband's."

"That is my point exactly. Springer is not your normal choice of TV. In fact you usually tell me that those shows are depressing."

"Actually I find them refreshing. There are people worse off than I."

"Worse off than you?" Mark pulled a chair up to the bed and it reminded me of being visited by a therapist. This led to my next sarcastic remark.

"You need a notebook to go with that?"

Chapter 3

"What?"

"With your sudden interest in my choice of words regarding Jerry Springer."

"My interest is in my mate and why she has suddenly fallen from exercising to binging and watching bad TV." Mark released a deep sigh, the one that lets me know he's worried about me and my sanity. "Also, why my wife suddenly thinks she needs to watch rednecks fight in order to feel better about her life."

"It was that or Oprah."

"So why not Oprah then? She usually has inspiring messages."

"Yeah, it was on how some person with a disability overcame it to climb a mountain or some sh**."

"You're cursing too. Hon, I think you need to call your doctor." Mark got up and began to gather up the bags of chips and candy.

"Oh, for goodness sake! I'm having a bad spell. It's not like I'm going to slit my wrists or something." I brought my legs to my chest and glared at him. Not only had he turned off the TV, now he was pacing about the room gathering up my snacks. I hated these talks and at the moment I felt like I hated him. How dare he decide when I'd been in bed too long? Why did he think it was up to him whether or not I ate junk food? He wasn't my father and I was grown woman. Mark paused at my mention of suicide and looked at me with worry.

"You've been thinking about that too, then?" I felt like screaming at him and instead snickered.

"No. It'd be too much of a mess to clean up."

"You'd be dead. And I would have to clean up," he remarked leaving the room momentarily to dump the trash and hide my snacks.

"And where would that get me? It wouldn't finish the laundry or clean the house!" I yelled. Mark walked back in with a stunned look. I stared at his eyebrows to avoid looking in his eyes. I knew I sounded ridiculous.

"That makes no sense and is downright depressing."

"This house is very depressing," I agreed.

"You're depressed because the house is a mess?" Men can be so difficult.

"No! I'm depressed because," I stopped. Did he just get me to admit to depression? I felt tears welling up in my eyes. It must have been frustration. I didn't want to talk about my feelings. I wanted to eat my chips and find out who fathered the baby of a 500 pound woman who used the f-word at least twice in each sentence.

Mark sat down silently on the edge of the bed. He just looked at me while I absently wondered how much of our lives were spent in the bedroom. I never felt it was fair to our son, Stephan, if I took over the living room when I felt this way. Our bedroom had become my private sanctuary since my diagnosis. I pondered how many days of the past four years had been spent in this one room. Not outside in the garden. Not out with friends. Just living in one room. I lost it. A few tears slid down my cheeks and then, when Mark wrapped his arms about me, and I fell into giant sobs. The kind that shake you all over and make you gasp for air.

"I don't know what to do!" I wailed into his shoulder.

"Shh, Hon. We'll get through this. We have before."

"But I'm already on so many drugs and what if a new one doesn't work? Or it takes six weeks for it to work? I don't feel like I can hold up anymore. I can't keep up with the house and Stephan. I'm not doing anything except making every-one miserable. Maybe I shouldn't be here." I sobbed more and Mark held on tighter.

"Tomorrow, I'll call the doctor and we'll see what we can do. In the meantime you are a wonderful mother. Even if you just watch TV with Stephan or pat him on the head, you never really neglect him. Besides you have a debilitating disease. You can't always be superwoman. Honestly, you shouldn't even try. That's what gets you into this. You need to accept who you are."

"That's just it. Who I am, is LAME!" I wailed, sounding an awful lot like a teenager. Mark giggled against me and the rumbling in his chest was comforting.

"You're not lame. You're just dealing with some bad fatigue and depression," he replied letting me lean away some as he ran his hands through my hair. He knows the hair thing al-ways calms me.

"But that's the point. How do we know if it's fatigue, or de-pression or just a relapse? There are so many things that can cause this and they are all linked to MS!" I pushed away to unload my nose into a pile of tissue next to the bed. I'd had a few crying spells earlier in the week but I knew they were all caused by sappy movies. "It could be my MS medication caus-ing this. It could be fatigue. It could just be having MS itself. How do we treat that? I don't know what to do!"

"Babe, you're thinking too hard," Mark replied sympatheti-cally.

"Oh? And what's the worst that's going to happen? I'll burn a few more holes in my brain from thinking too hard." Mark rolled his eyes at my snippy reply.

"Didn't we just get past the part where you growl at me?" My hackles went up. One thing about depressed people is that it is very easy to piss them off. We know we're down and we need to get up, but damned if we wouldn't rather pull you down instead.

"We'll get over my griping when you get finished lecturing." I grabbed the tissue box and vigorously blew my nose. Mark made a harrumphing noise and ran a hand through his hair.

"I think you need drugs," he muttered. I tossed the box across the room letting it land with a thud and threw my hands into the air. Being overly dramatic is also an added benefit of being in an "I don't care" mood.

"Finally a suggestion that I agree with! Get me a drink." Mark looked scandalized and I laughed.

"You've got to be kidding. I was talking about anti-depressants! Besides it's daylight."

"Pull the shades and we'll pretend it's evening." I said suggestively. Mark now seriously looked concerned and before he had a chance to dial the cops for a 51-50 (woman gone mad) I relinquished my one amusement for the day, now that he had turned off Springer. "All right. Tomorrow I will call my primary and get a Prozac rocket." I flashed a fake grin, because honestly almost all my grins at this point were either fake or sarcastic in nature. I truly was a bitch when I felt low.

"Prozac rocket?" he asked. I nodded. "That's a new one for you. You should write that down."

"Don't worry love. I will." I fluffed the pillows behind my back and felt the beginnings of a cry-headache. The one I always get after a good cry. It feels like a tight band around my skull at the same time that my eyes feel dry and made of dust. I lay back against the pillows feeling spent. Mark must have noticed that my claws were sheathed and that I was worn out. He tucked a blanket around me and handed me back the remote.

"You will call, won't you?" He kissed my forehead. I sighed. I didn't want another pill added to my regimen.

"Yes. I will call. First thing." With the promise, he left me in peace and I turned Springer back on. The credits were rolling and someone was tackling the huge woman. "Damn." I looked over at the rolodex on my desk. "Well, things really could be worse."

So to make a depressing story shorter, I called. Got my rocket, and blasted my butt back to normal. Well, Lorna normal that is. I also learned that when I begin to watch Springer with avid interest and my bed is filled with crumbs that it is time to look at depression. I also realize that while a pill may have helped me once, there are times when my depression was lifted by a change of diet, and -insert groan here- a bit of fresh air and exercise.

An Ode to Sleeping Pills

(This was written before the birth of my second son, Aidan in September 2004. Since then, sleep is no longer an option in this household.)

I had many sleepless nights during my diagnosis of Multiple Sclerosis, but I thought normal sleep would return after the diagnosis. It hasn't. Okay, it is not every night that I wake up near dawn, but that is mainly thanks to pharmaceuticals and not inner peace. Here is a short story about my quest for a good night's sleep.

The reason for this waking, for me anyway, is usually the same. I have to pee. If I do not wake immediately, I'm sure to experience a shifting in my dreams from running about flower filled meadows to looking for the nearest bathroom. I have endured some seriously twisted bathroom dreams. I will spare you. Eventually, I wake and wobble to the bathroom. No matter how hard I try and I try, sitting there thinking, "Don't wake up. Keep eyes closed. Do not wake up." I always fail. By the time I'm finished in the bathroom, I'm awake.

Then comes the endless minutes of shifting and rolling, fluffing and pulling, to make myself comfortable in the bed. With random leg cramps, tingling and back pain, this is often a long series of thrashing movements followed by Mark threatening to move me onto the couch if I don't cease and desist. I usually take more of the covers in retaliation. Most people with MS experience insomnia due to these random body pains. I, like many others, have medicines to help with these pains and while they can make a person drowsy, they do not put you to sleep.

But now it's time to try to get back to sleep while ignoring the ramblings of my mind. The experts say that when a person sleeps, the dreams they have are simply the mind running the defragmenter program. That all of life's stressors past and present are jumbled into some odd images that filter through the brain while we sleep, in order to make some sense of it all. So while our brain is solving problems and ditching old files, we dream about giant chickens riding with us in an elevator that goes sideways. Go figure.

Yet after waking enough to use the restroom, it feels to me that this defrag program is still running. So I get the wide awake version of my brain filtering stress. First the "shoulds" kick in. These are a group of guilt-ridden stressors. Everyone has them, but I think women and mothers rank a bit higher on the list. I should do more with my son. I should pitch in more around the house. I should write more. I should do more with MS MOMS.

Next, I get the random worries that usually filter through as we fall into sleep at the beginning of the evening. Is it garbage day tomorrow? Did Mark put out the trash? Did I pay the electric bill? Will the neurologist listen to me at my appointment this month? Then comes the deeper, hidden guilt and regrets, the ones that only come out in nightmares: every single memory I had hoped to delete from my memory banks, everything I feel I have screwed up starting with my childhood and running to my most current temper tantrum when I yelled at my son. A therapist once told me that I needed to feel these events and then let them go. I let the therapist go.

However, it is not my personal neurosis that concerns me. I've been neurotic for years and slept just fine. It is my inability to shut them off and go back to sleep. This led me to the conclusion that besides needing to pee constantly and being hard pressed to get my body comfortable in bed, my MS has also somehow broken my on/off switch. Since my MS is 75% cognitive and 25% physical—it truly is ALL in my head—it makes sense to me that something like sleeping would be screwed up. I already put the milk away in the cupboard and flip the bathroom light to flush the toilet. Why not attack my peace of mind at night? MS in the past five years has slowly wreacked havoc on my attention and memory.

At first I tried to avoid any sort of napping during the day so that I would be so exhausted that, come bed time, I would pass out and not wake until the sun hit my face. Next, I tried staying up very late until I was unable to avoid falling asleep. However, I just awoke at the same time as I do every other morning and spent the day short on sleep. I cut the caffeine. I cut back on alcohol. I exercised, and although it helped with falling asleep, I could not stay asleep.

So I turned to Benadryl. Most over the counter sleep aids like Tylenol PM and Nytol are made of the same ingredients as Benadryl. I'm figuring the drug companies saw a big opportunity when people on antihistamines kept drifting off to sleep at their desks during the day. Okay you don't drift. One minute you are thinking about your plans for the next day and then it IS the next day. Unfortunately, I get Benadryl hangovers, I feel funky all day long. And I don't mean in the 70s sense of funk. I walk about not thoroughly refreshed but in a daze. I also built up a tolerance to it. If I take a full dose, two pills, I spend the next day drowsy and sluggish. If I take one, it barely affects me at all. So Benadryl is only good every once in a great while, or if I've been stung by a bee.

I brought this problem to my primary care doctor, whom I am thinking of signing up for sainthood. He understands MS and is not afraid of my questions and ideas. At only my second visit with him, he instantly gave me a prescription for Ambien, a sleeping pill. When the bottle tells you not to make any plans for eight hours, it isn't kidding. Not only do you not drift off into sleep, you don't remember when it hit. It truly is the 8-hour, how-the-hell-did-I-get-on-the-bathroom-floor-so-you-can-rest-medicine. Ambien has been the closest thing to a good night's sleep in a long time. After you've been shot by the Ambien tranquilizer gun, you awaken feeling refreshed, revived, and curious about what you were doing in the 30 minutes before the pill kicked in.

Now the down side. These sleeping pills can become habit forming, so you cannot take them every night. Well, no duh! If it puts you to sleep and helps you stay asleep, no wonder they are addictive. In today's world, getting a good eight hours of sleep is like finding a truly silent place and that's worth fighting for. Silence is golden. It's also round and marked "Ambien." So some days I awaken like Sleeping Beauty and others I drag out of bed groaning like a grumpy zombie. If they ever find a way to make them non-addictive, I'll be the first in line.

Vertigo

Vertigo when described by health pages is a false sensation of motion or spinning that leads to dizziness and discomfort. Discomfort. Uh-huh. In all actuality, when my MS vertigo kicked in, it was a room spinning, cannot open eyes or walk, horrible nausea, profuse vomiting, how the heck did I end up in the hospital, kind of discomfort. My mother properly named this "You can't die fast enough," after she had a run in herself with vertigo on a cruise.

There are two kinds of vertigo: peripheral and central. Peripheral occurs if there is a problem in the vestibular labyrinth (semicircular canals), the portion of the inner ear that controls balance. This type of vertigo can be mild (discomfort) to as bad as mine was (debilitating). The harsher kind of peripheral vertigo is usually caused by a virus. Central vertigo is caused by an abnormality in the brain, particularly in the brainstem or cerebellum. Guess which one I had?

Up until that one morning when I woke up with the room spinning, I had always thought of MS vertigo as a sort-of dizzy spell. I never imagined that it could end a person up in the hospital. I apologize to anyone who has experienced this before and has dealt with people unknowingly thinking it was a bout of the spins.

To accurately describe the spinning feeling one must either imagine what it felt like as a child when you used to spin until you fell down laughing. Either that or recall the last time you were falling down drunk and holding the world down. Take that brief feeling that dissipated if you just gave it a few moments, or a night of good sleep and imagine it not going away.

Sure I had some warning signs before my brain lost the off button for the spins. Sure, I had been feeling a bit off-balance and dizzy for a day or so, and figured I was just stressed. Because I was going through a period of intense stress and it was a time when I was not taking good care of my health. The night I fell asleep with the room moving, I figured some rest would make everything go away. Wrong.

When I first opened my eyes and the walls were swimming, I closed them again and rolled to my side. In the past, this usually took away any dizzy spells I had. But this time the spinning didn't stop. I recall telling Mark that the room was moving. Next thing I knew, I was holding on to the toilet with closed eyes, praying that I would pass out. Because honestly, when I have my head in a toilet I'd rather be unconscious and not know about it. Wouldn't you?

I kept thinking that if I sat up straight, my head would adjust itself. This is again how I dealt with dizziness in the past. Let me remind you this type of vertigo is NOT simple dizziness. Mark soothed me by saying it would pass.

Next time I cracked my eyes open, I was surrounded by some handsome men in blue shirts. I wondered if I had finally passed out, until I recalled that I was in my night-gown and that I was propped against the bathroom door. Closing my eyes again, I prayed I WAS asleep because whether I had been waylaid by vertigo or not, I still had some pride. The last thing I wanted was to be in front of strangers barely dressed. Mark had called 911.

"It gets better if you lay completely flat." I cracked open my eyes to find a woman with red hair smiling down at me. From what I could pick up of the surroundings, the metal color to the walls and the rocking, we were in an ambulance. Either that or my dream had taken a worse turn and I was floating down a river in a metal sardine can. The spinning feeling had lessened just enough for me to crack my eyes again.

"I thought I had to sit up," I croaked. The car took a turn quickly and I closed my eyes again groaning.

"That is everyone's instinct, to sit up and right themselves but lying flat is better."

"My husband?"

"He's right behind us."

It was amazing how strong the urge to open my eyes was. As they shifted me from ambulance, to the ER, and then to the hospital bed I felt helpless and without my sight. I wanted to know what was going on and what they were doing, but I could not keep my eyes open long enough. I only got to peek and received flashes, making the whole scene more like a music video, with quick, choppy images.

What seemed to me like moments later I felt well enough to peer through my eyelashes and get a better idea of my situation. Mark was beside me reading and instantly got up and took my hand. I was shivering and asked for a blanket. In fact my body was now quaking so hard I felt I needed at least 50 pounds of blankets to stop the moving.

"It's the fluids from the IV. They are making you cold from the inside out." I heard Mark say this as he pushed back the curtains and left the area. I figured he was getting more blankets.

Of course I had an IV. I don't think you can leave the ER without your free IV! Apparently they had administered some medication for vertigo along with Valium and now were hydrating me. At least I could peek at the scene and I no longer felt like

I needed to have a bowl sitting on my lap, just in case. Now I felt that if I lay flat and never moved again, I would be set for life. Mark came back in and piled some blankets on me.

"Are you feeling any better?"

"I don't want to move ever again," I whispered.

"Wow! You need a breath mint!" Leave it to my dear husband to bring something like this up. I think he knew he was safe bluntly commenting on the state of my breath while I lay motionless in the emergency room. I couldn't sit up and smack him with the pillow, I couldn't even yell. Instead, I opened one eye as wide as I could and glared.

"Do you think that could have something to do with vomiting all morning?" I remarked, having to close my eye back down. I wondered if the scowl on my face was just as threatening as if I had both eyes on him.

"You look like an angry Cyclops, Love," Mark laughed softly. Obviously, my scowl wasn't working.

"Do you have a mint?" I asked softly. There was something about how my body felt that told me if I raised my voice it would equate movement and set my spin cycle off again.

"Nope," Mark replied cheerfully.

"Then why tell me about my breath?" I clenched my hands under the blanket. In my state, it did not dawn on me that Mark was distracting me from the shaking of my body and my overall unpleasant situation. I just wanted to throttle him. The doctor came in before I could finish my plan on how to inflict pain on Mark without moving. When the doctor asked me if I could open my eyes, I peeked at him. He was glancing at my chart.

"So you have Multiple Sclerosis?" he asked. Mark answered for me and I grunted in ascent.

The doctor asked a range of questions all the while leaning close to my face and shining a light in my eyes. Apparently this was to see if I had nystagmus. While this sounded like something about stags with mussed hair, it was instead a problem with my eyes. Nystagmus is the rapid movement of the eyes either horizontally, vertically, or round and round. When a person experiences vertigo there eyes can go wiggy like this. Apparently mine were vibrating horizontally. Mark later said it was rather odd to watch.

I kept wishing the doctor would get out of my face because I did not want to breathe on him. After all, according to my sweet husband, I had "death breath." Apparently doctors are made of stronger stuff than husbands are, because he did not comment on my horrendous breath nor get out my face. After being in my face for so long studying me, I began to wonder if the doc was having eye trouble. Then he gave his prognosis.

Unfortunately, for the brave doctor who could withstand death breath and still smile, he said the one thing I hate hearing. (Second, of course, to "You look fine.") Either it was an ear infection, or it "Could just be your MS." Mark asked about both cases and their treatment, while I squeezed my eyes shut again, exhausted from having them open through the exam. For an infection, antibiotics. For my MS, treatment was some Valium, motion sickness meds and bed rest.

This is otherwise known as the "Here. Have some pills and go live with it" plan of treatment.

"If it is her MS," Mark asked, "how long would it take to go away?"

The answer? "I'm not sure. Go ask your neurologist," pronounced the doctor. This, in my mind, is the MS equivalent of "Go ask your Dad." Because when I cannot be sure of an answer to a question of Stephan's, I always send him to the answer specialist: Dad.

Next, the doctor cheerfully informed me that he would be back in an hour to do some shifting positions with me that would help "right the crystals in my ear," just in case it was an inner-ear problem. He also used the words "minor discomfort" and my pulse, which was being monitored, shot up a few notches. I could hear Mark trying not to find this amusing in the background somewhere. Mark knew very well that I believed anytime a doctor mentioned discomfort it meant "great pain." In this case I got to look forward to minor pain, which was exactly what my husband was being.

I decided to forgive the doctor for his "It could be MS. I dunno," comment. After all, he had withstood my breathing on him and so far seemed truly sympathetic to my pain. ER doctors can be very kind, especially when your eyes are bouncing back and forth in your head. Before I knew it, my hero was back and asking me to sit up.

After sitting up, I no longer liked him. He grabbed my head in his hands and asked me to lean to the right as if I was falling off the table. Mark got to help just in case, I listed too far to port. Now, hanging half way off the table with the room starting its spin, I decided that not only did I not like the man, I was beginning to envision others with vertigo storming his house with pitchforks and torches. That was until he had me hang off backwards. Now I was not envisioning, but planning, his imminent death. If you have ever experienced vertigo, you would be right there with me, torches lit.

All of this, which left me lying back on the bed clinging to Mark's arm with my eyes tightly, closed hoping against all feeling that I did not spew. The test was to see if it made my eyes go wiggy even more. Surely this shifting would help him to make a more concrete diagnosis? Not really. He said he was thinking it was more likely my MS, because my voice was slightly slurring and I seemed extra weak on the quick exam he had given me before he got in my face with the bright light. However, it could all be an ear infection.

I was told the shifting would help if it was my ear, and was sent home loaded with Valium and my prescription for Anti-Vert and more Valium. I spent more than a few days in bed. Then because the vertigo had eased, I tried getting out of bed. I am not good at bed rest and began making Mark's life a bit hellish as I tried to get back on my computer, about the house on weak legs, while slightly dizzy, and slurring. It just didn't work.

My father came to the rescue when Mark told him about how much trouble I was having. He brought me a nice looking, black padded, wheelchair. When I asked where he got the chair, he joked about living in a park with seniors. "Someone always kicks the bucket and leaves their stuff." I had forgotten. Dad always said what is on his mind and saw this as a rescue mission. I was thrilled at his forethought and a bit creeped about the possibilities of where my chair came from. Dad reassured me that some people have surgeries and when they are done with the chair they also put them in the clubhouse at his place. Still, have you ever been to Disneyland and ridden in the haunted mansion? Know how when you leave in that spinning chair you see a ghost sitting on your lap? It felt like that. Kind of creepy. But hey, I had asked the question.

I got in the chair and Mark began two weeks of pushing me everywhere, when I could handle the movement. There was an up side to temporarily being in a wheelchair. No, it is not all the polite people, because half the time they bump into you because they don't "see you down there." The up side for me was dressing up. You see, thanks to my vertigo and the necessity for a wheelchair, I got to wear my long colorful skirts and my high-heeled suede boots. These I had bought for my trip to London. But that was the trip where I had my first relapse. These clothes had been shoved to the back of my closet because I could not get around in them safely. Now, with Mark in charge of my transportation, I felt free to wear whatever I wanted. I only had to worry about it if I had to get up, or if it would be uncomfortable to sit in.

Within a month, I was feeing more like myself. The room did not spin, I could actually type again without using a speech-recognition program that barely recognized my speech. (When I cursed at it, it came back with something about a "cheese heist.") After recovering, I could walk straight. Well sort-of, but I never walked all that straight before Vertigo.

But when the Vertigo left, I had to say good-bye to my boots and my flowing skirts. I didn't miss the vertigo and in fact was very careful (read paranoid) about anything that would spin me about for years to come. I stayed off rides at the local fair for at least two years, afraid the spinning would make the nightmare start all over again. Over all, Vertigo truly was a "You can't die fast enough" experience. The recovery made me very dependent on those around me and proved, yet again, how much Mark and my father loved me. But I came away from the flare-up knowing that now even Vertigo could not unbalance my spirit.

Pregnancy with MS
(Or There's a Rabbit in my Laundry Room.)

There are a few things I have learned about getting pregnant with Multiple Sclerosis. First, you need to quit all your medications. Second you need to be totally unprepared, and third you need a rabbit to show up at your house. This was how my pregnancy with my second son, Aidan began.

On the New Year, I quit all of my medications. (I don't suggest anyone follow my lead and do this without consulting a doctor first.) I went through some nasty withdrawal, and in retrospect, it was very foolish of me to do this without a medical OK. But I felt that I had hit a wall with my treatment. It seemed every time I had a twitch, doctors were adding on a new drug.

After my diagnosis, I would have been thrilled to have doctors responding so quickly to my symptoms. Five years later, it began to feel that as soon as someone saw the letters "MS" on my file, they decided that no testing was needed. All I needed was a pill. I felt sluggish and no longer had a clear view of my condition. When something did happen, I was no longer sure if it was my MS or a side effect of one of my many medications. Besides, no one knew what the real, drug free Lorna was like.

That January, drug-free Lorna was a heinous bitch. With a rabbit.

I have always had a soft spot for animals. Even after my diagnosis, I brought home everything with fur, feathers, and scales. I'm sure a psychologist would have an idea as to why I did this, but this particular January, we were down to just a few cats. Had I suddenly become anti-pet? Word must have spread through the animal kingdom that we had an opening for a stray, because in late January while I was tromping through the house, going through withdrawal, and being generally irritable, a rabbit showed up in our laundry room.

The white lop huddled next to the washing machine looking pathetic and cute all at once. Knowing it had to be someone's pet, we put a large dog carrier, left over from one of my animal obsessions, in front of where it was hiding, and it instantly hopped in. When, days later, it became obvious that no-one was going to claim the rabbit, and that both Mark and Stephan were thrilled with it, he became our permanent visitor. We even occasionally let him out to hop about the living room. By the first week of February, I felt better, had renewed energy, and the rabbit had eaten through our satellite TV cables.

I had commented in an email to my family that a rabbit was a sign of fertility and a new beginning, but in general I had quit paying attention to signs. January had been a difficult month and I was really favoring realism. It was after all just a lost pet. I should have known that in *my* life nothing is as it seems.

When the second week of February came, my energy continued to increase and my MS symptoms seemed non-existent. But Mark brought up the point that my irritability, which we originally blamed on medication withdrawal, had amplified. I blamed it on PMS. He, in return, politely pointed out that PMS did not last for three weeks. It had to be something else.

I had never experienced a man telling me to go buy a pregnancy test, but that is just what Mark did.. We had discussed trying to have a child after I got drug-free, and in shape, so I thought it wouldn't hurt to find out when I was ovulating. In fact, I had snuck out only days before to purchase an ovulation kit Now the ovulation kit sat unopened and I was tearing into a pregnancy test to prove Mark wrong. The idea of using the pregnancy test before the ovulation kit felt very much like the chicken before the egg.

The kit had two tests. I quickly scanned the instructions making sure they had not changed since the last time I had bought one in a state of panic over a late period. Mark must have gone off his rocker, I thought as I dipped the stick into the cup. We had not been very sexual during my detox, after all it is hard to get close to a prickly woman, and I didn't get pregnant at the drop of a hat. Or at the drop of a rabbit, rather. I washed my hands and prepared to leave the bathroom to find our egg timer (no pun intended) because the test said it took five minutes. I glanced at the test stick on my way out and did a double take. It had only been about 40 seconds!

Thinking my Optic Neuritis had flared, I covered one eye and then another to check for double vision. Nope. There were two distinct lines in separate windows. I grabbed the instructions and read them again. One line was the control line, a nice shade of pink, and the other, the test strip which detected the HCG hormone. I looked at the test line. It was purple! I covered my scream, half joy, and half terror, and ran from the bathroom faster than I had moved in years.

Mark was in the living room taking a business call when I slid into the kitchen looking like Tom Cruise from Risky Business. He was pretty involved with the headset on and pacing the floor as he talked. Mark glanced up at me and then went on talking, likely thinking I was creating, or attending to, some household disaster. When I stopped my slide against the kitchen table and bounded into the living room, he paused in his discussion and looked at me again. For about two seconds, then went back to talking. I considered screaming at him, but instead joined him in pacing our living room until he was off the phone. Mark looked at me strangely, not knowing I had taken the test, and I broke the silence with the best thing I could think of saying.

"I'll do another test in a few hours."

After the initial shock, and Mark pointing out that he was right, we rejoiced. However for me, it was short lived. Soon after excitedly sharing the news my doubts set in. Would my MS harm the baby? Would my having Multiple Sclerosis make me a high risk pregnancy? Would I be able to handle the stress of carrying and then delivering a baby? What would happen to my symptoms? How would I handle nine months without any help from medications, if my symptoms did flare? I lay awake nights switching between feelings of joy and fear.

As usual, I turned to the message board of MS MOMS and the rest of the internet to find out information on MS and pregnancy. I also bought the only book out there devoted to MS and pregnancy, a book I had often recommended to others from its Amazon.com ratings. I only made it through the first few chapters before asking my mother to finish reading it and tell me if there was any helpful advice.

I handed the book over because it was depressing. While the comments from other parents with MS in the book may have been helpful and honest insight before I got pregnant, reading it while pregnant was horrifying. One lady even stated that if she had known how hard it would be after the baby was born, she would never have gotten pregnant! With my fears and concerns, this was not something I wanted to hear. Thankfully my mom did take the book and relayed the pertinent information to me. She is a wonderful filter.

As it turned out, my MS did not harm the baby. I experienced a blissful 9 months of remission. This is common for many women with MS. In pregnancy, the body naturally suppresses the immune system so that it does not attack the fetus. This is why you often hear advice to keep sick people away from pregnant women. Doctors and scientists speculate that it is this suppression of the immune system that leads most women with MS to have a period of remission during pregnancy. (Since our immune systems are thought to be whacky.) For me, this theory was very true. MS-wise I felt better than I had in years.

In the view of my obstetrician, having multiple sclerosis did not make me a high risk pregnancy. I was also informed that later in the pregnancy, if I was struck down by a large relapse, steroids could be used. Thankfully, I never needed them. I never needed anything stronger than Tylenol for the usual aches and pains of pregnancy. The stress of carrying Aidan was only a burden to pelvic muscles which rearranged themselves to adjust for the extra weight.

Not being treated as if my MS was detrimental to my pregnancy, helped me to enjoy it. (As much as you can enjoy mood swings, morning sickness, and backache.) When I went for my prenatal visits I sat in the waiting room with the other expectant mothers feeling just like them. If I slurred my speech or dropped words they assumed I wasn't getting sleep because of my belly. I never worried about walking funny, because we all walked funny!

I will admit I still had worries, but they usually ran along the same lines as other moms-to-be. Such as: Will he have 10 fingers? What if I've forgotten how to be a mom? Or What if he has two heads? (Come on, all of us have had nightmares close to that while pregnant.)

MS was such a miniscule part of my pregnancy that I abandoned any ideas of writing a book on it. What would there be to tell? I felt great? I finally felt MS-free for the first time in 5 years? It would have been a very short book. My pregnancy with Aidan, in regards to MS, was completely uneventful. That's not to say the pregnancy was without incident.

Near the end of the pregnancy, I was diagnosed with gestational diabetes and had to use insulin. The main thing that annoyed me to no end about gestational diabetes was the diet. I have always viewed pregnancy as the one time women do not have to worry about eating the vegetables on our plate. (Especially the ones we secretly dislike as much as our kids do.) I'm not saying pregnancy is a ticket to eat whatever you want, but well…yes I am! We should be free to make some less than perfect choices along with our daily intake of greens.

Obviously my diabetic nurse did not agree with my view that ice cream was a good source of calcium and chocolate sauce was essential for keeping pregnant mothers calm. My body didn't agree either and I ended up taking insulin shots each morning. Thanks to my previous experience with MS, I was the only woman in the "How to Take Shots" class that was smiling and saying, "What a tiny needle!" The other women looked ready to choke me.

As it turned out, the regular ultrasounds and heart rate testing the doctors did because of the diabetes, helped to show when Aidan was ready to come out. After a 3-D ultrasound, which Mark had gifted me with, showed that Aidan appeared much further along than he should be, my OB ordered a test of her own. She didn't trust "those 3-D people." Because of her mistrust of the 3-D ultrasound we discovered, not only was Aidan big, but my amniotic fluid was low. Mark kept teasing me that I was quart low and I had to agree at 37 weeks pregnant I felt as big as a truck.

When Aidan began showing signs of fetal distress and my amniotic fluid remained low, I was sent off to the hospital. Did I blame my MS? No. When they decided to check me in for labor induction and delivery that very evening, I fretted more about not having the nursery ready than any imminent danger. My theory was that it wouldn't do Aidan any good if my pulse shot sky high and I went waddling about the maternity ward predicting the end of days.

Having been sent to the ER by my MS on many occasions I'd developed a warped view of what warranted panic. So I settled myself in and busied myself talking calmly to the nurses. Mark was sent home to pack a bag which I had not prepared yet. The nurses helped me pass the time by betting on what we thought Mark would forget to pack.

Once Mark was back and praised by the nurses for being a man who remembered everything his wife requested, the real contractions kicked in. There was no time to freak out. The next thing we knew, I was being shaved for a possible emergency cesarean. Aidan's heart rate was erratic and if he didn't chill out they were going to pull him out. Mark paced frantically while I took deep breaths and envisioned a perfect baby. I had my fears and doubts but reminded myself that now was not the time to panic. I put my faith in God and the hospital staff and knew that whatever needed to be done would be done. I also needed to reserve my strength for whatever lay ahead whether it was a caesarean or pushing.

I wasn't quite sure why I felt calmer than I had in previous emergency situations. Maybe I was loopy with labor, because when the nurse told me to forget the cesarean because they were going to insert a large tube inside me to flush the womb with fluid, called amnioinfusion, I didn't shout, "You're what? You have got to be kidding me!" This would have been my reaction at any other time. I mean first I' was a quart low and now we were going to use a hose to refill my water! Aidan was lucky we didn't decide to name him Ford or Chevy.

However complicated the birth seemed to get, I did not panic. Ok I panicked, but in the form of my blood pressure getting low while I took deep breaths. I've seen mother cats do this in labor, especially when there's trouble. They lay back, get droopy-eyed, and purr. I didn't purr but I wasn't grabbing Mark by the collar blaming him for my condition either. Mark was the one who paced the floor and growled at everyone. I just held on and prayed. Until my epidural came.

Then I lost my cool. I mean, come on, the last two times a needle got close to my back I ended up with a headache and a diagnosis of MS. When the anesthesiologist asked me to sit up and hunch over, I could hardly move. The nurse helped pull me into a sitting position and with all the tubing I now had hanging from parts of my body, this was not a comfortable thing to do. Not to mention it brought on contractions. So when the anesthesiologist asked me to bend myself in half, so he could stick a needle in my back, I lost it. "I have a huge bump which stops me from bending in half, called a baby," I hissed. I swear he laughed, but I couldn't turn and check.

Once the epidural took effect, the labor ended quickly with a normal vaginal delivery of my healthy 7lb 9oz, chubby, pink, bundle of boy. Do I ever think that my MS was the cause of my difficulties, NO! In retrospect, I believe my various experiences with MS and all its scary symptoms is what helped me to remain calm! Somehow labor pains pale in comparison to spinal taps and vertigo. Where my MS did come into play was during the post-partum period.

When Aidan was about three weeks old, the gray clouds of doubt began to circle as I noticed that I had spent an entire morning rubbing at my eye. Yes, I had some numb spots on my legs and still got tired rather quickly, but I had blamed all that on the epidural and recovery from giving birth. A cloudy eye however was not going to be ignored. And neither was Mark who noticed I was rubbing my eye again. So off to my neurologist it was. Well, I hadn't seen the neuro in awhile. Maybe he missed me. I ended up on steroids, diagnosis MS flare-up.

In the end, the hardest part of being pregnant with MS was

giving up the nine months of remission. I had energy and generally felt like the old me. Nine months is a long time and it was easy to get used to living without my MS. After Aidan's birth, I tried for awhile to blame everything that could be MS on the stress of giving birth. You know, I'm still numb because. I couldn't bring myself to admit that my MS had not magically disappeared and that it was still a part of me.

My point is that I "knew" I could have a relapse, but I didn't really know how to prepare myself. I had people lined up for the first few weeks after Aidan came home, but never used them, because I felt great. (Like a woman who has just been treated like a truck and then run over by one, but overall pretty good.) It was month 2 and 3 after Aidan was born, that were the hardest.

I didn't want to think about my MS. Surely my problems in both of those months could have been attributed to the stress of a new baby. I didn't want to face the truth because it meant I had to go back to being what I felt was "less than." Yet I couldn't deny ending up on steroids twice in the first 3 months of Aidan's life.

I was forced to make a decision. Accept it and enjoy my new son or flounder in self pity? Sure I wallowed in a few pints of ice cream. I also lay in bed for a day or two, but I knew if I stayed there I would miss a lot. Aidan's first grin for example. By the time he was five months, things were approaching normal. But it was a new normal, like everything else with MS. The rules keep changing. It was up to me to fight it or fly with it.

Looking back over this pregnancy story I can admit that after having Aidan, I experienced more than one flare-up. But it would not stop me from having another child. In fact, it was nowhere near as bad as I imagined it might be. I do not think that pregnancy should be avoided because of a *chance* of relapse. Living life with MS means always living with the chance of a relapse. Some women give birth and are just fine. Worn out but fine. Some, like me, experience a period of flare-up or relapse before settling into their "new normal."

Like most pregnancy books for the average woman say: "It takes nine months (for your body) to get that way, it takes nine months to undo it." I think Multiple Sclerosis and the postpartum period should be regarded with the same attitude. The first weeks or months may be very hard, but with time, things will find their balance. Besides, we get such a lovely parting gift!

CHAPTER FOUR

Shark oil

Steroids

Steroids. In the past visions of body builders and disgraced athletes came to mind when someone said "steroids." Nowadays the image of Terminator is replaced by thoughts of corticosteroids and their use in Multiple Sclerosis and other immune responses such as allergies. I know more about steroids now, but it is definitely one of those areas I wish I could have remained blissfully ignorant in.

First of all (and no, I'm not going to turn this into a lengthy scientific paper on steroids, I just feel compelled to insert a few facts before I begin the rant), steroids are broken up into two groups anabolic and corticosteroids. Anabolic steroids are the kinds which have been used illegally by bodybuilders and athletes in the past. Corticosteroids are the kind most usually prescribed to decrease inflammatory responses. (If you ask me, after the mood swings I experienced, they INCREASE inflammatory responses.)

In Multiple Sclerosis corticosteroids are the most common medicines prescribed when a person is having a relapse or flare-up to speed recovery -and deflate swollen things such as nerves and lesions-. (Don't quote me on that because every doctor has different reasons for prescribing.) Since my dx in 1999 I had heard many MSers online talk about needing IV steroids etc for their relapses but never once do I recall anyone complaining overmuch about them. Thus, when I was prescribed steroids for my optic neuritis in January, I wasn't a bit concerned.

Because I had not come to him as soon as my eye began to trouble me, my neurologist did not order IV steroids for my optic neuritis, but instead prescribed a course of Prednisone tablets. Sometime in the 1950's a movie was made about a man taking Prednisone. He subsequently goes crazy and kills his wife. According to the story about this movie (which could all be medical urban legend), people became afraid to take Prednisone for fear they would go insane. Going mad was not something my neuro mentioned when prescribing the medication. He simply told me he wasn't going to use IV because I hadn't "come in from the start."(As you know from the earlier installment, I wasn't ready to blame my MS and that was why I hadn't rushed to my neuro when my eye went nuts.) Speaking of nuts, let's get back to my steroid reaction when I began taking Prednisone.

Within the first 24 hours I noticed a change in my sleep. I had trouble going to sleep the first night and awoke at 5am the next morning, not a wreck but instead with my head whirling full of ideas and motivation. For me, who lacks motivation unless it involves cute animals and shopping, this was a rather invigorating experience. I was charged, awake, and ready for anything! I didn't drag myself to the gym; I wanted to go more than once a day!

Along with this energy came a sudden fearlessness that allowed me to tell people what I REALLY thought about them. Maybe it's because cortisol is a natural hormone like adrenalin produced by the adrenal gland that this sudden "pumped" attitude came about. Adrenaline is the hormone released in the flight of fight response to stress. It's what pumps our body up in order to get us ready for hauling/kicking butt. Whatever it was, things I'd kept under my hat for years were now easily aired out. Being passive-aggressive, this ballsy attitude was completely anti-Lorna. Whereas before I always avoided that rush of adrenaline signaling confrontation, I now relished in it. In fact I was practically begging for someone to piss me off so I could fight. (And this was only day two.)

Then things got worse. (Like you didn't see this coming.) I went from looking for fights to perceiving even the slightest thing as an attack. I became jealous, suspicious, and down right surly. For the record my husband would like me to use the term, Heinous Psycho B**ch. For once, I'd have to agree with him. I cried at the drop of a hat, screamed the next. I wanted to call people up and confront them about things that went down years ago. I found myself thinking, now where is that girl from the 7th grade's number? I've got a few words for her! After a full 48 hours of shorting my sleep and overworking my body at the gym, because I felt great, I began to slide downhill even faster.

Hormonally it sort of felt like being 13 all over again. (Except let's make that a 13 year old boy!) I would holler at Mark for something I thought was simply the worst thing in the world, whether it be leaving dirty dishes in the sink or the seat up, and then I would flounce out of the room punctuating my anger by slamming the door. After that I would throw myself face first on the bed and sob as if the world were falling apart. Yeah, it was just like being 13 again. My arguments made little sense, my emotions were overblown, and I thought I could take on the world. (Add in trying to limit my fighting to when my son was not home or explaining to him why Mommy was slamming doors and my brain was completely fried.)

While my son was at school on the third day, after another big fight involving my suspicious idea that the whole world was attempting to annoy me on purpose, (yeah I was certifiable) I drove off in a tantrum. I don't drive much to begin with, which is a whole other story, but Lorna driving off angry, NEVER happens. This was also most likely, the stupidest and most dangerous thing I could do at that point. When I came home to find Mark sitting in the bedroom talking in hushed tones to our roommate, I was able to realize that not only had I scared everyone, but this was simply not ME. (But I wasn't ready to admit it to anyone yet. I am genetically a woman after all, and we never admit wrong doing.)

So I pretended to ignore the fact that Mark looked haggard and went flouncing into the room as if I'd just gone shopping. I couldn't however turn a blind eye to the fact that both he and my roommate were talking to me in soft voices with wide eyes as if I was some wild animal and they were trying to lure me into a corner with a tranq-gun. That would have really worked too! Why don't they hand you the steroids AND a tranquilizer gun for your spouse? Hey we could do that for PMS! You know, if the chocolate runs out and you start foaming at the mouth your mate can simply shoot a dart into your backside and you'll sleep it off.

I went into my walk-in closet and had another good cry. Mark tip-toed in and knelt beside me, offering kind words and reassurance. He rocked me while I wailed that I was having a nervous breakdown and that maybe all my enemies were right and I WAS insane. In a calm tone Mark guaranteed me that while I was a bit "different" from most women, I was most assuredly not loony. We both agreed that it was quite possible the steroids were causing this severe fluctuation in moods and he made me promise not to drive until I was off the steroids. While he pet my hair and told me how much he loved me, I fought between wanting his comfort and wanting to arm wrestle him. I still had 8 days left at 3 pills a day. I knew I wasn't going to make it, so I called the neuro.

When calling I was quite sure they were going to think I WAS nuts, because I expected to hear that people did fine on Prednisone and that once again it was simply Lorna's odd reactions to medication. Instead, the office assistant K, the sweetest woman in the world, told me "Oh this happens all the time!" I thought, gee why didn't he warn me about the tendency for some people to react to Prednisone by going totally whacko? They switched me to Decadron and because I needed to taper off, I spent the next 2-3 weeks being, the new and improved, Heinous Bitch Lite (without any added preservatives or psychoses!)

Since this delightful journey into the wonders of feeling like a real MAN -because all I wanted to do was exercise, fight, and *you know*- I have found that people who get IV steroids don't have such a big reaction. Some have no side-effects at all. Overall most get pumped and then crash after the 3 days are up. It was suggested to me that maybe taking pills over a longer stretch like I did, is what caused such nasty side effects. (Or I have a heinous bitch inside me dying to get out?) Whatever the reason, next time I would rather 3 days of an IV, complete with big crash, then go through the Hell I went through. (I'm positive now that when Dante wrote about Hell, he left off a level called Steroid.)

However, I can completely understand how people can be pumped up on their own feelings of righteousness and make horrible mistakes. Because that's how the energy felt, righteous. I was suddenly God and boy were there some people I wanted to smite. While I have to admit that feeling unafraid and full of energy was quite freeing, the dark side of my reaction to steroids was an enslavement of another sort. I now have to admit feeling sympathy for men. The constant feelings of being attacked or being ready for an attack were tiring in their own right. The empathy that is so much a part of who I am was completely shut down. I not only frightened Mark but myself as well. I was short on sleep, hyper, and edgy. Edgy like a wolverine, not edgy like a sharp haircut.

When Mommy went off her steroids and peace came back to the land, my family released a collective sigh of relief. I went back to lying on the floor instead of waxing it, and the feeling of tense, electric energy that had run through the house was once again replaced with the usual scattered, mellow aura. I, on the other hand, felt the crash profoundly. Sure I had told people off and wouldn't let Mark get any sleep, but the quiet time I had at 5 a.m. was something I had come to enjoy. I would watch the news with a cup of coffee while I penned down ideas for the day in the silent house. I had felt vibrant and in-charge, albeit in a sort-of mad-scientist fashion.

Oh yes! My eye, the cause of this completely nutty scenario, did get somewhat better. I'm still experiencing difficulties months later, but I'm told that is how Optic Neuritis runs. My family survived my nasty temper, sobbing, and the "let's go for a 2 mile hike" energy at dawn, all in one piece. I've now learned that if my Guide to Pills states, "may cause mood swings," that it's an understatement just like when your doctor says, "you may feel some discomfort." The mood swings, were more like "complete alteration of personality," and the doctor's "discomfort" usually equals extreme pain.

As I look back on it now, although I felt I had more Oomph, nothing truly got done, except damage. So next time I'll opt for the IV and be more like Frankenstein's monster than Mrs. Hyde.

Addiction

I'm going to start with a little disclaimer. This "rant" is not for everyone with MS, nor does it necessarily reflect the average MS patient. I am focusing this discussion on medications. Why would this not be a topic for everyone with MS? Because this topic tends to relate more to those of us with MS who take many medications daily. Within these medications are bound to be a few that are technically considered "addictive." While I think Ben and Jerry's ice cream should be labeled addictive, that's another topic.

Junkie. Addict. The Webster definition is: "to devote or surrender oneself to something habitually." Doesn't sound too bad. It could sound rather responsible, like cleaning house every Sunday. Then it continued, "or excessively." Well, there goes the cleaning defense. Then Webster went on to give me a clearer description, "to cause a person to become physiologically dependent upon a drug." I admit it. I looked up physiologically next. But only because I wanted to be sure I knew what it meant in layman's terms. Physiologically means "dealing with the body."

Therefore, I concluded, an addict is a person whose body is dependent upon a drug. Well, gee! Then insulin dependent diabetics are addicts. Right? If I consider not taking my shots this usually means my MS gets worse, and then my body is dependent on them to not eat its own brain. That makes me instantly an addict, as well. Of course eating brains is something more psychologically wrong I think, but you can't put your white cells in group therapy. So I am dependent upon my MS therapy to keep my body from falling apart. And this whole time I thought being an addict was a bad thing. My son thinks being an addict means you're that small space above the living room, but that has absolutely nothing to do with this article.

The literal definition of addict is not my problem. What is stuck in my craw, is how do I decide when the medicine I take is something I require to combat my MS and to enhance my quality of life, or when it is something I'm addicted to? Quality of life is a common term when speaking about how to make a MSer's life more comfortable. For example, if a cane will help me get out more often then it is enhancing my "quality of life." I have never felt comfortable using my cane, but I'm off topic. Although not all symptom-relieving medications used in MS are addicting, there are many that cause eyebrows to raise and good ole addiction paranoia to set in. For example pain killers, muscle relaxants, and anything whose generic name ends in "am." Lorazepam, Clonezapam, and Diazepam are a few.

Some doctors, bless their souls, are actually interested in working with their MS patients instead of instantly labeling them as addicts when they ask for these "baaad" medications. They believe that the main goal when treating MS, besides putting the person on one of the medications to slow the progression of MS, is to help the patient have the highest quality of life. Anything that can ease the MS sufferer's symptoms, so that they can go about their life, is okay in their book. There are even MSers out there who have been prescribed, or are using, marijuana for their MS. Shh. This may be an extreme view, but I see no harm in that. Yes, they run a risk by using an illegal substance, but I'm not going to call the Feds on them, would you? Heck, if smoking a chicken foot eased some of the more painful symptoms that hit me at times; vertigo, facial pain, and spasms, pass the foot! By the way, no need to hide your chickens, I thankfully have prescriptions that deal with my painful symptoms. And no, they are not green, leafy prescriptions.

My issue though, is not about the use of marijuana in MS. My ire starts when the doctor believes they'd rather let a patient suffer and avoid the "risk" of addiction than prescribe. This sort of issue happened to me a few years ago with diazepam, commonly known as Valium. Much to my surprise, Valium is one of the best things to prescribe a person for vertigo. Valium can make you loopy but it can also help when you're loop-da-loopy. Go figure. When I was struck by vertigo, otherwise known as, "You can't die fast enough," back in February of 2002, I was prescribed Antivert and Valium.

During my follow-up care with my neurologist, I was given more Valium. I am quite aware that when my vertigo kicks in again, as it does if I don't take care of myself and my symptoms flare-up, my neuro will probably give me more Valium. Besides, we aren't talking truckloads of Valium. This is a prescription that I take daily for maybe 3-5 days until the room quits spinning when I lift my head or try to walk. We are talking short-term usage. But just the mention of the word to anyone, other than my neurologist, caused suspicion. I learned this when a few months after the vertigo, I asked my old primary care physician, who was always in contact with my neuro, if she would be able to give me an "as needed" prescription. Instead, I got a lecture!

"It's addictive," she told me in hushed tones.

"Yes, and in my case there are times when it is necessary," I replied. I explained to her about my vertigo and how I would rather have something on hand, maybe four pills, in case it struck again so that I would not have to go through the rush to the hospital in an ambulance again. Besides why do they always have to start you on an IV? And why hook me up to all those machines? Do the EMTs have a secret bet running on who can get one patient hooked up to the most tubing? When she continued to go on and on about addiction, I got irritated.

"It's not like I'm snorting it," I said sarcastically. She didn't think that was funny. In retrospect, getting on her case was probably not the best way to go, but I was annoyed. First off, how would a small prescription of four pills start me on the road of a pill-popping junkie? Secondly, it felt like she was already insinuating that, even by asking, I had some sort of problem. Besides, if I did have a problem, I'd be buying the stuff online illegally from Mexico instead of going through the trouble of a prescription. I knew people with MS who were taking loads of technically "addictive" substances and were never harassed about "addiction." It made me wonder if that was why some were taking the back road to management of their symptoms. The leafy, green back road or the Mexican express.

It also made me question the basis doctors used for judging addiction versus necessary medication. What makes them decide whether or not you're in need or just a junkie? Is it age? At the time I was on the young end of MS at 26. Is it length of diagnosis? I had only been diagnosed for three years. Maybe it is based on how the patient looks? I didn't appear sick or off-balance at the time. Therefore, I must have been asking for it in order to sell on the street to fund my nefarious plans for world domination. Or possibly to buy the leafy green stuff.
What decides it? Where is the line? Moreover, when a person is diagnosed with a debilitating, life-long disease, don't the rules change a bit? I guess in that doctor's case it did not matter. She had to be right, I had to be wrong. I'm not ranting because I attempted to get some "hard core drugs" and got turned down. My neurologist, thank God, understands my condition. I'm irritated because I wonder how many other people are being refused medications because of the "chance" that they may become addicted.

From what I was able to find regarding the practice of prescribing controlled substances, especially in the case of pain, there is a big line drawn in the sand. Some doctors are on one side, rating quality of life over chance of addiction, and the others believe you find alternatives to these controlled or addictive substances. Yes, and usually their patients smoke something and then get a massage. It appears this is one of those never ending moral dilemmas for doctors. Do you give the person a potentially addictive substance so that they can have a better quality of life, or do you refuse and give them some lame alternative because of the chance that in the long run they might become physiologically dependent? Gee, tough choice.

You can see where I stand. Alternative practices can be helpful for many things and I have used them in the management of some of my symptoms in the past. But, in the case of the more life-altering symptoms of MS, spasms, pain, and vertigo, I believe that unless the doctor is going to hire an acupuncturist and a masseuse to hang out in my living room, they had better give me a prescription that always works.

So I can sell it on the street to fund my plans for world domination.

Herbivores: MS and Herbs

Like most people, for most of my life I took what the doctor prescribed. Except for that time in college. He didn't prescribe that, but I didn't inhale. Who did? Until my first summer after my diagnosis, the closest experience I had with herbal healing was Chamomile tea for tummy aches. Being newly diagnosed, my neurologist seemed reluctant to prescribe any medications for symptom relief. I don't know why. Maybe it was just a newly diagnosed thing. You get the meds after you go through a year or so of hazing. So that summer, I turned my hobby of planting herbs into a study. If the doctor wasn't going to help me, could those little plants? And no, they weren't the ones with seven pointy leaves.

When I turned my attention to herbal healing, I was not interested in supplements or pills, but in the old fashioned use of teas, baths, and ointments. In my opinion, drinking a cup of herb tea was not putting me at risk for any drug interaction. I looked at it as a natural way to combat my symptoms. Besides many of these ideas were old family remedies anyhow, so how could my mother-in-law be wrong? I just imagine many of you thinking of your own mother-in-law and getting worried for my safety at this point.

However, as I learned, many herbs do have strong interactions with over the counter and prescribed medications. So, just to be safe, I got a book on drug/herb interactions and checked every herb before I added it to my regimen. The only prescription medication I was taking at the time was Copaxone for slowing the progression of my MS. According to the handout that comes with the shots, you know the one with fine print smaller than fine print, there did not appear to be any herbal interaction problems. Then it dawned on me that most likely this was because no one had tried this yet and that I might be the first person to become ill from a disastrous mixture of Copaxone and catnip. (She drank what?) Therefore, I double-checked with my books and websites.

When educating myself, it was amazing how many interactions could occur between herbs and conventional medicines. One theme I quickly noticed was that if I was taking a prescription for the same effect I wanted from the herb, it would probably have a bad interaction. One example would be Xanax (prescription) versus kava (herb) for anxiety. It reminded me of some young siblings I know. They are made from the same parents, yet try to kill each other on a constant basis. Helpful books and websites for herb/drug interactions are listed at the end of this article.

After satisfying myself that I would not be the first person to be hospitalized for mixing catnip with MS shots, I went on to learn that many herbal store employees are just that: employees. The have no clue about MS. This was just fine, because most of the herbs I was going to use were growing right outside my window. However, it pays to be aware that they will often try to sell an herb or supplement to enhance what they think is a weak immune system. I began to feel that the next time someone handed me a bottle of Echinacea to pump up my immune system, I was going to need something more than chamomile not to throttle them. That would have only served to get me expelled from my favorite herbal store. They promote peace and surely bouncing a bottle of pills off the turned back of an employee would be seen as an act of violence, not peacemaking. So, as usual, I kept my tongue and my reactions to myself and bought my catnip and chamomile with a calm smile.

Bad interactions with medications and people aside, let's move on to how I used four different herbs in helping with my MS symptoms. Remember these were very mild herbs and not supplements, otherwise I might have gone the kava route. Trust me no herb, or pill for that matter, can magically take your symptoms away forever. Oh, if it only could! But the following ideas and recipes may help you, as they helped me. Those of us with MS know that every bit of assistance we can get leads us closer to a fuller, richer life.

I mainly used the herbs to steep and make a tea or to infuse a bath. A BATH?! Yes, a bath. Most people with MS know that hot water can make aggravate our symptoms. Something about our damaged nerve coats getting swollen and irritated. Like most of us women before our period. Temperature safe baths steeped with infused herbs have been my savior many times in the past. I'm not saying lukewarm because that usually means near freezing to me. Teas, on the other hand, are faster and easier to prepare than baths, and can taste delicious as well. Note that I said "can taste delicious." Some herbs are harder to swallow than others are. Finally, oils, lotions, and poultices can be made with some herbs and put directly on the skin. These applications work wonders for sore muscles, cuts, and burns.

Herbs listed here can be bought at most local nurseries during the spring and summer season. I don't suggest you get them off the streets from a guy in a trench coat. You may already have some of these teas in your home. Here are some of the ideas and recipes I used for helping with different MS symptoms.

CATNIP
Yes, that same herb you buy for your cats. It may make them roll on the floor in psychedelic bliss and then race around the house as if their tail was on fire, but it has a calming affect on humans. Catnip works as an anti-spasmodic and mild sedative. However, catnip does not leave you feeling like you just popped a Valium. If you are taking Valium or any other sedative or muscle relaxant, I wouldn't add catnip into the mix. While

it isn't as potent as medications like Valium, it does take a bit of the edge off. Everyone is different, just as MS is different for everyone. Reactions to catnip will vary greatly. Some of you may feel very loose and others may think, "Why am I drinking this green stuff?"

Directions:
You can buy natural catnip already dried at either a pet store or a natural food store. Just hope that while at the pet store they don't ask if it is for your cat when you don't have a cat. Try explaining that one.

If you have a living catnip plant, take some of the leaves and let them dry. You can use them fresh as well, but remember to double up if using fresh leaves. If you have cats, try to keep them from rummaging in the plant. (Good luck!) When they bruise the leaves, the scent is released and that will only bring them to heights of gloriously destructive ecstasy. (And attract more cats!) Bruising of the leaf takes some of the medicinal juice out of the plant, as well. You'll have to choose between your stress or the cat's fix?

To make catnip tea, boil some water and then pour the hot water over some of the catnip leaves. Usually for an infusion I use two teaspoons of fresh catnip per cup of boiling water. Do not boil the catnip itself as it looses its precious oils. The recommended limit is three cups a day.

For bathing, I have found it easy to make a catnip bath and some tea at the same time. Take a coffee filter and brace it over a plain jar. That way, you don't have to tolerate leaves floating in your bath or tea. For a stronger infusion, mix the hot water and the catnip and then strain it. But don't boil. Once you have done this, let it sit and steep for about ten minutes. The water will turn green. Pour the green brew into your bath or cup and enjoy! Catnip tea is minty, but you may need extra sweetening to your taste. I like my tea strong and green!

My uses for MS:

Helped with spastic muscles, anxiety, and relaxing. Catnip has helped me greatly when I have been over-stressed or anxious. I also found it relaxed cramped muscles, too.

Warnings and interactions:
Catnip is considered non-toxic, however, beware of any potentially dangerous add-on depressant interactions when you combine catnip with drugs in any of the following depressant drug classes: alcohol, anti-anxiety (Xanax, Ativan), anticholinergics (Ditropan), anticonvulsants (Klonipin, Neurontin, Depakote, Valium), antidepressants (Paxil, Zoloft, Prozac, Wellbutrin), antihistamines (Benadryl, Allerga, Claritin), muscle relaxants (Robaxin, Soma, Flexeril), antihypersenitives (Tenex, Catapres), antipsychotics (Mellaril, Risperdal, Lithium), narcotic analgesics (Demerol, any form of Codeine, Percodan), or sedatives (ProSom, Doral, Dalamane, and nonprescription sleep-aids such as Tylenol PM.) Five years later looking over this list, I would guess that just ruled out most of us for catnip nipping.

Catnip can cause stomach upset if too much is ingested. I recommend you check with your health care provider before using catnip or any other herbs for yourself, if you are pregnant or nursing, and if you are over the age of 65. If you have MS and are using the bath, remember to take temperature smart baths. Becoming overheated can make your symptoms worse and ruin your relaxation time.

CHAMOMILE:
Yes, the stomach tea. Chamomile is one of the best selling herbs on the market. It has similar anti-spasmodic qualities to the catnip, a pleasant aroma, and tastes great. Chamomile has been known to help promote sleep, ease menstrual cramps, and stomach upset, plus it may help with ulcers. Chamomile is a main ingredient in those sleepy time and nighttime teas you bought and never used. They're sitting in your cupboard right

now. But I bet you never thought of tossing the tea bags into your tub! Yes, I have done this but you'll get a much better effect if you buy the plant or dried flowers and make an infusion.

Directions:
The part of chamomile that is used for teas and baths is the little white flower with the yellow center. If you have ever had chamomile tea, when you smell the flowers you will recognize the scent immediately.

Two or three teaspoons of chamomile flowers per cup of boiling water make a wonderful, relaxing, tea. Limit is three cups per day. To avoid floating weeds in your cup, use the straining idea I suggested above. For commercial preparations follow the instructions on the box. For my needs nowadays I generally use store bought. Less mess and no fuss. For a bath, tie the flowers together in a coffee filter or a cloth baggy and run it under the water as the tub fills.

As with the catnip, you can find the live plant at any nursery or get the dried flowers at a natural food store. Chamomile is easy. For those of you who would rather take the easy way out and not be accused of odd potion making in your kitchen, go to any nearby grocery store and buy the tea. But we know it's already in your cupboard, behind the baking soda. If you're looking for a simple way to relax before bedtime, store bought teas will do the trick. However for most people with MS sometimes you need a bit more kick. This is where making the infusions or baths comes in.

Relaxing chamomile baths may help calm tension and muscles. As with catnip, you can steep the flowers in jars of hot water and then, after ten minutes, pour the water into the bath. The water will turn yellow. So you know have a choice between green water and yellow water. Which one do you think will make the kids freak out first?

My uses for MS:
Anti-anxiety, helping promote sleep, and for its anti-spasmodic qualities like Catnip. You can mix catnip and chamomile. Many of those store-bought teas use both herbs in their ingredients. The combination can be used for an extra soothing bath. When mixing herbs, remember to use smaller quantities of each. If you have stomach problems, chamomile is also a digestive aid and may help with ulcers.

Warnings and interactions:
To my dismay, after using chamomile for quite some time, I read that British researchers found that chamomile's uncanny ability to help with infections is due to its ability to stimulate the immune system's white blood cells. This is of course not good news for those of us with MS. However the tests were done involving chamomile oil directly applied to the skin, not baths, or tea. It is not known how much stimulation is done and this seems to be a secondary characteristic in the herb's medicinal abilities. For me, it became a fight between a relaxing tea before bed or the paranoia of creating more raging white cells.
In response, I tend to reach for catnip before chamomile, but still see no harm in a little yellow tea before bed. Possible interactions are lesser than with catnip. Be wary of chamomile if you are allergic to ragweed or dandelion. There have been some pretty nasty reactions in people with this allergy who have taken chamomile. Also there are possible interactions between Chamomile and Heparin (a blood thinner), Trental (pentoxicfylline), and Coumadin (warfarin, an anticoagulant).

Once again, it is a good idea to check with your doctor before using catnip or any other herbs for yourself, if you are pregnant or nursing, and if you are over the age of 65. If you experience any stomach upset, nausea, or vomiting, stop use immediately.

RED PEPPER
Yes, red pepper. It has been found to be an invaluable herb

not only for clearing out your sinuses and causing your friends to laugh at you when you make that face after eating it, but for its analgesic properties when it comes to helping pain. While many doctors out there like to say, "There is no pain with MS," this is entirely untrue. I learned this first hand when I began to have what is called Trigeminal neuralgia. Otherwise known as, "It feels like someone is poking your face repeatedly with a needle."

Directions:
Most people aren't going to have a red pepper plant. Heck, I don't. But the herb is readily available again at both natural food stores and the grocery store. In fact, it's probably in the cupboard right next to the chamomile tea and baking soda. Most likely you will find it listed as cayenne pepper. This is a bit of a misnomer since only a tiny fraction of the U.S. red pepper supply comes from places like Cayenne in French Guiana. But if you can't find it listed under red pepper it's usually being called Cayenne.

Red pepper can be made into an infusion for digestion, but in the case of its use for MS symptoms, we're going to grab the vegetable oil. This is to the right of the baking soda. Use 1/8 to 1/2 *teaspoon*. I can't stress teaspoon enough. Lord help you if you make this with a half tablespoon. That's 1/8 to 1/2 tea-spoon of red pepper per cup or warm vegetable oil to make a nice balm. This can be rubbed on to the area of pain. This area was, for me, my face. That makes my next warning particularly hilarious.

Warning and interactions:
Do not get in eyes. Think pepper spray. This becomes exceed-ingly difficult when rubbing the stuff on your face. When the red pepper balm was used in patients with cluster headaches the biggest side effects were watering eyes and burning nos-trils. However the pain did subside. Be very careful about touch-ing your eyes or nose after using the balm. If you can stand a

bit of eye watering and nostril warmth, this balm can help. Now if you're chronic pain is in another area, you're in luck, as long as you don't wipe your eyes after rubbing it on. Red pepper has a possible harmful interaction with Theophylline (a once commonly used treatment for Asthma, also sometimes used in sleep apnea cases) and a possible helpful interaction with Non-Steroidal Anti-Inflammatory Drugs (NSAIDs) like Aleve, Advil, Naproxen, Aspirin, Vioxx, and Celebrex, to name a few. Since this is a possible helpful interaction, I'm guessing you rub on the red pepper and take your Aleve. But remember, you don't want this in your eyes.

My uses for MS:
Red pepper balm was used for Trigeminal Neuralgia, head-aches, and anything else cramping or throbbing. If you have facial neuralgia, please use this with caution or simply skip it. As I found it was very difficult to not get it too close to my eyes and while my pain eased, my eyes looked and felt like I'd been in a fight with an onion.

MINT
Whether it is spearmint or peppermint, the mints have always been successful at lifting my spirits just from their invigorating scent. When using the mints, I tend to use peppermint more than any other because of its flavor. Peppermint just tastes better. Another wonderful aspect of peppermint is that it is FDA approved as a cold remedy. Mints have helped immensely when I am sick with a cold or stuffed up from allergies. A strong cup of peppermint tea or even a soak in the bath helps clear my sinuses and chest. Peppermint is also a stomach soother.

Growing mint is very easy. It's keeping it from growing every-where that is difficult. Mint is one of those creeping plants that loves sending itself all over the yard via runners that snake out all around the plants taking over whatever it can. If you don't want a plant whose main goal in the garden is to throttle your chamomile, you can just go buy the stuff at a grocery store as a pre-packaged tea. Natural food stores often carry dried mint leaves, that can be used as well, but you must buy a special strainer, use a homemade one like the one I mentioned earlier, or submit yourself to floaty things in your tea.

Mints have always been one my favorites since I was a little girl. My mother used to have mint growing along side of the house. Every time I smell that crisp scent I am transported back to those summer days of lazing around the yard with my mother. Maybe mint brings back some memories for you, too.

Directions:
To prepare a mint tea (if you do not already have the tea bags), use one to two teaspoons of dried mint per cup of boiling water. Steep for about ten minutes. You can drink up to three cups a day, but more may cause stomach upset or diarrhea.

To make an infusion bath with mint, use few handfuls of the dried or fresh leaves and place them in a cloth bag or a coffee filter tied at the top with a twisty tie, then let the water run over it. Another way to do this is to boil some water and then drop the handfuls in the water, letting it steep for about 15 minutes and then straining the water. You can then take the infusion you have made and add it to your bath. Once again like catnip, which is in the family of mints, the water will turn green.

My uses for MS:
The best use for mint with my symptoms was helping to give me a bit of a boost when I was horribly fatigued. It did not give me extra energy, but the scent of mint is very invigorating and helped me on days when I just wanted to feel more awake, even if only 20 minutes or so. Even though it is not listed as one of peppermint's traits in the herbal books, peppermint has been used widely by those involved in aroma therapy to lift spirits and raise energy. I believe it has something to do with the "fresh" and "clean" scent that mint gives off.

Warnings and interactions:
Peppermint and spearmint are included in the FDA's list of herbs generally regarded as safe. Possible drug interactions for peppermint are with Antipsychotic agents and NSAIDs, which means you can't use mint with your pepper rub and Advil party. Since there was no listing for other mints, I would think the same goes for spearmint.

Spearmints should be used in medicinal amounts and try to get approval from your doctor or research any possible interactions carefully. I recommend that you do not use mints if you are pregnant, nursing, or over the age of 65. If you experience any stomach upset or diarrhea, stop using immediately and inform your doctor. Mints may be used in children, but they should be diluted and discussed with the pediatrician first.

Catnip, chamomile, mints, and red pepper were great help to me during that summer without symptom relief medication. If a person with MS finds themselves in this situation, they may wish to try some of these ideas. For all of us, these four herbs can come in handy as a safe, simple way to help relax. After you make sure that you are not using something that can interact badly with your current medications. However, I don't profess that these are miracle cures, but I do believe that a gentle cup of tea or a soak in the tub couldn't hurt.

If you are interested in herbal help, look into these books which I used. If you get advice from an herbal shop or decide on a treatment yourself, it is always recommended to either research the herbs for interactions and side-effects or check with your doctor before you start treatment.

REFERENCES

Books
Bratman, Steven, M.D. and Harkness, Richard, Pharm., FASCP. 2000. *The Natural Pharmacist Drug-Herb-Vitamin Interactions Bible.* California: Prima Health a division of Prima Publishing.

Castleman, Michael. 1995. *The Healing Herbs: The Ultimate Guide to the Curative Power of Nature's Medicines.* New York: Bantam Books.

Weiss, Gaea and Weiss, Shandor. 1992. *Growing and Using the Healing Herbs.*
New York: Wings Books.

Blose, Nora and Cusick, Dawn. 1993. *Herb Drying Handbook.* Brussels: Sterling Books. (This book includes complete instructions for microwave drying.)

Bremness, Lesley. 1998. *The Complete Book of Herbs, A Practical Guide to Growing and Using Herbs.* New York: Penguin Books.

Websites
About.com Healthy Herbs http://healthyherbs.about.com/cs/drugsearch/ Accessed February 25, 2005
(This is about the only website you need because it is a list all the websites for checking drug/herb interactions. You can also get information about herbs and their healing properties here as well.)

Snake Oil

Here is another touchy subject I feel just screams to be poked at. The Multiple Sclerosis CURE. I'm going to state for the record right now that the only CURE for MS is to not have it. Or maybe I can go so far as to callously state that the only cure is death. Because as far as I know, at this writing, there is no medical cure for MS. There are a lot of things in the works. Medical trials are going on as we speak, but last I heard, those who decide our fate, a.k.a. the medical profession, still have not figured out why MS happens. So, how could they have a cure? That said, many people out there claim to have been cured of their MS. Whenever I find this written on my MS MOMS message board I am hard-pressed to not roll my eyes or at least sigh for the poor soul who has been sucked in by some cock-eyed theory.

While many people think that snake oil vendors disappeared with the 1907 Pure Food and Drug Act, I know that they are still alive and well. All you have to do is get diagnosed with a disease like Multiple Sclerosis and they come slithering out of the cracks ready to sell you a cure for "only $19.95 a month with a free tote bag!" More confusing is the fact that I can be alerted to this cure by trusted friends and family. Harder still is when a fellow MSer has tried this pill, diet, cream, fish-dance, and found relief from all symptoms. MS is relapsing-remitting for most of us, which means they could also have experienced a remission and their symptoms were going to disappear any-how. But they go so far as to claim they have been cured. "And why shouldn't you try it too?" they ask.

This is always difficult to deal with. Mainly because it is one of those damned if I do, damned if I don't, situations. How do I tell a person who is currently free of symptoms, that I simply do not believe whale blubber pills are the cure for MS? Worse yet, how do I explain to them that it was posted on the trusted site www.quackwatch.com, created simply for the purpose of weeding out these phonies, that the blubber pill man was arrested in his mother's basement?

If I do, I am not only insinuating that their cure is something akin to snake oil, I am also telling them they are not cured. This not only makes me cold-hearted, it also makes me a faithless pessimist who keeps her eyes closed to possibility. I like to think that pessimists are simply optimists with experience.

But I am not closed to all possibility. I am merely opposed to snake oil and quacks. Tell me, why do they label these fake medicines and those who peddle them with animal references? How did they take the sound a duck makes and turn it into the definition of a fraudulent doctor? In my defense, I have tried alternative therapies from herbal remedies to going off all medications and using only diet, exercise, and faith to handle my MS. So I am not untried in the area of alternative therapies. In my mind there is a big difference between snake oils and most CAMs.

CAM or Complimentary Alternative Medicine is the use and practice of therapies or diagnostic techniques that may not be part of any current Western health care system, culture, or society. In 1991 congress gave funds for the creation of the Office of *Alternative Medicine at the National Institute of Health* (NIH). Since this time, much research and many studies have occurred. These findings are often published in journals relevant to CAM such as Alternative Therapies, Alternative Therapies in Clinical Practice, and Journal of Alternative and Complementary Therapies. However, the quality of information is assorted, and little scientific evidence is offered for claims made.

I have used alternative therapies in the past, ranging from herbs like catnip to calm muscles to aroma-therapy with lavender oil to ease headaches. Today I still turn to chamomile for its soothing effects before bed or to ease a stomachache. None of these treatments are approved by the FDA, which requires years of study and instead are mainly old family remedies. As I wrote in another article, when I could not get symptom relief from my neurologist, I turned to herbal therapy for symptom relief. While not as fast nor as potent as pharmaceuticals, they were effective. So I am not opposed to alternative therapies as much as I am to "cure-alls." I never expected a soak in catnip or a tincture of chamomile to cure my MS.

It irritates and saddens me that, more often than not, people pushing alternative therapies are expecting a patient to use their product instead of their regular MS medications, as opposed to supplementing them. (Always make sure when supplementing with any CAM that it does not conflict with your regular medication.) The mindset I often run into is not one of "take this along with your medications to help." Instead, it is usually "Traditional medicine prescribed by a doctor is harmful, and you have to quit taking everything and start drinking blended seaweed." Whenever I am told of a "cure" or a therapy that requires me to stop taking everything else and adopt what adds up to be a completely different mindset, I get skeptical. Nothing better illustrates this than the last time I attended a New Age convention.

In the past, my husband and I attended and sometimes had a booth at these alternative shows. They had vendors ranging from tarot card and aura readers to the vitamin and alternative treatment sellers. On instinct, I avoided the booths containing these treatments but instead headed for a massage or a fun tarot reading. But of course during a reading, the subject of my Multiple Sclerosis came up. No, a woman wearing a beaded head wrap did not suddenly look at me and say "you have MS!" I told her. Readings are always fun and to me, good readers are more therapist than psychic. I believe that sometimes the best insight into a situation can come from a stranger, whether they are holding a deck of cards or next to you on a bus. Anyhow, after my reading, this friendly woman decided she just had to escort me personally to the vitamin booth. Because vitamins sound healthy and promote a sense of trust in the consumer, I am assuming. After all, vitamins are sold at our grocery stores, so they can't be bad for us.

Since my husband was busy talking business with the promoter of the show, I let her drag me across the crowded room. I knew I wasn't going to buy anything, but I somehow felt obligated to the tarot reader, and didn't see any harm in letting her do her best to "guide" me to help for my MS. She introduced me to the older lady behind the table and then was off, back to her table.

The vitamin seller, let's call her Betty, instantly went into her pitch about what I should take for my MS. I tried to look naive as she explained to me that shark oil was my best bet. Betty had sold this to a woman in a wheelchair who now walked daily. While I was deciding whether or not to ask if the MS survivor walked nightly as well as daily, Betty slapped a $70 bottle into my hand. I looked at the pills that according to directions would only last two weeks and then at Betty who was giving the grand finale by telling me these would "build up my immune system, because people with MS have compromised immune systems."

"Actually, it's the opposite. Our systems are over-pumped and need to be tuned down. That is why we are warned not to take supplements like Echinacea," I said softly. Betty made a tsking sound that older motherly women make when they are about to tell you that you're wrong. She patted my arm and shook her head.

"Oh, you're wrong dear. Your immune system is not working hard enough. You need these pills."

"What about my other medications? The ones prescribed to me by a doctor?"

"After these, you won't need those. In fact many of those medications are dreadfully harmful to the body. They are full of toxins." She gave me a smile that was supposed to convey she was going to let me in on a secret, then added "My sister has MS. She took these and has not been afflicted since." Really? Why didn't you mention that right off Betty? Give me those oily capsules! I put the pills down and pulled my arm away slowly, feeling like she might blow a gasket if I disagreed further. Let's just say my sixth sense was going off. Taking the easy way out, as opposed to attempting to educate Betty via argument, I told her that I left my purse at home and my husband had all the money, so I needed to go discuss it with him. I left her table rapidly. How many people had bought these expensive pills? How many had quit all of their prescribed medications and turned over their pocket books to people like Betty in the hopes of finding a cure?

Thankfully, unlike the days of the historical snake-oil vendor, these non-prescription medicines are more carefully regulated. As I learned, some are helpful as supplements or when conventional medical treatment is unavailable. I don't believe that a cup of tea hurts anyone. (Except maybe Socrates, but that was something completely different.) Alternative therapies are usually safe and I encourage people to explore them. But only after they do some research by using sites like Quack Watch and making sure that the supplement, whether vitamin or herb, will not interact with current prescription medicines. The broadly termed "alternative medicines" can include treatments ranging from dubious to bizarre. Often they can lead a person down a dangerous road guided by people who are uninformed or simply out to make a buck. As I discovered at the New Age convention, it wasn't snake oil being peddled it was shark oil!

REFERENCES

Spencer, John W., PhD. and Jacobs, Joseph J., M.D., M.B.A. 1999. *Complementary Alternative Medicine, An Evidence Based Approach.* St.Louis: Mosby, Inc. A division of Harcourt Publishing

CHAPTER FIVE

My Two Sense

The Summer Blues and Beating the Heat

Below I have combined an article that ran in the MS MOMS newsletter in 2000 and a rant from summer 2004. Together they show how heat can get you down, and also some tips on how to deal with heat.

I hate summer now. I never used to hate summertime in fact, as a child, I loved swimming and being out of school. Multiple Sclerosis has essentially ruined summertime for me. Well that isn't completely true. I just can't live in it like I used to. The main reason summertime and my multiple sclerosis don't mix is heat. Therefore, if I lived in England, summertime would be wondrous. But here in sunny California, summer is hot. Most years I now spend a majority of the summer months inside as opposed to getting a swimsuit tan at the pool.

When it gets hot I, like the delicate flower I am, wilt. All right so I'm not a delicate flower and I tend to do a better impression of the wicked witch of the west screeching "I'm melting!" but that's beside the point. The point is heat makes my Multiple Sclerosis symptoms worse.

The reason heat has this effect on most people with MS is because an increase in body temperature further impairs the ability of our stripped (or demyelinated) nerves to conduct electrical impulses. Many of us have shorted our hairdryers by getting them overheated. Our cars even go kaput when they get too hot. This is similar to how heat affects MSers. When we get hot, we go kaput.

Whereas heat used to feel mildly unpleasant, it now has become unbearable. When first diagnosed, my main constant symptom was fatigue. So when I got hot, I did a wonderful impression of slug-woman. Now, five years later, many other areas of my body are affected by MS and the heat. When I get hot I get fatigued, my vision goes funny, sensations go haywire, my right leg does not want to work, and my cognitive problems come out in full force. Unfortunately, I'm a rather "well" looking 29-year-old lady and most people end up assuming that I'm staggering and slurring from one too many wine coolers. This is so unfair. Who grocery shops plastered at 10:00 a.m. anyhow?

Most MS literature tells me that once I'm cooled down, the temporary worsening of my symptoms will go away. Yeah. I recall many times that I've gotten too hot, wilted, and then after cooling down in my dark room, re-emerged as chipper as I was that morning. I also recall the time I saw a monkey driving a double-decker bus down Main Street. The whole idea that cooling down is all a person with MS needs to feel instantly 100% better is about as accurate as a blind man looking at a police line-up.

Sure, if I am overheated, the best thing to do is get cool. But I'm still shot for the day. I'm not going to bound from my room within 20 minutes ready to take on the world. I'm most likely going to play queen bee, shouting orders from my bed for the rest of the busy bees most of the afternoon. The downside to this is that I feel guilty the whole time, so I can't even enjoy being waited on. I have quickly learned that the longer I spend in the heat the longer my recuperating time is.

Getting cool and staying that way has become a big production for Mark and me. When I was diagnosed, our little home only had a swamp cooler with no central heating and air. Now we have a wonderful little air conditioner for the living room and one that fits in the bathroom window. With these two air conditioners running and a series of fans placed strategically throughout the house, I can keep reasonably cool. Mark, who is actually handier than most men I've encountered, installed a ceiling fan in the bedroom as well. He helped make our little farm house hospitable when the temperatures soared above 100 and gave me the chance to cool down.

The down side is that I created a prison for myself, albeit a cool one. Each year I have become more intolerant of the heat. So, I retreat to my bedroom turn the air on, close the shutters, and relax in my little, cool, dark room. Some days this retreating is relaxing. Other days, I become edgy and depressed. On bad days, it is like being the sick kid who sits at the window watching all of her friends play outside. I can see and hear my son playing outside in the sunlight but know that if I join him I am shot for the rest of the day. I do venture out on occasion, usually in the early morning or late evening. This summer schedule ends up making me feel like a vampire. I lay silently in my tomb-like room until night when I emerge to stalk the city. Going to a movie is nothing so dramatic but I do get to feeling something like a night creature when the only time I feel that I have energy is closer to 12:00 a.m. than 12:00 p.m.

Mark asked once why I was so opposed to staying inside where it's cool, since I never was the outdoorsy type. (Except when I was much younger and got any access to any body of water, and became part fish.) Whether or not I'd be outside in the sweltering heat if I didn't have MS doesn't matter. It is the fact that I can't choose to be outside that bothers me. I'd like to be able to plan a trip to the lake without thinking about how miserable I'm going to feel afterward.

Of course there are many steps I can take to beat the heat and be outside. But all of them require a will to be outside that is stronger than the misery I am going to deal with later. I can buy a neck cooler, put on light colored clothes and down three gallons of ice water to go hang out in the sun. However I am still going to be fatigued when I get home. No matter what people say, unless I was in a cool-suit from head to toe, I am still going to feel the effects of a 101 degree day.

Besides, and I know this is vain, I hate the idea of walking around with some device on, making me look like an alien Yes, I know I sound like a hypocrite because I advocate doing anything to spend more time with family and friends. However, I also advocate feeling as close to human as possible so that you do not lose yourself in MS. That said, below are some of my tips for beating the heat so you can enjoy some time outside in the summer. And not have to wear a space suit.

1.   Take some of your scarves or bandanas, get them wet and then put them in the freezer. These cold rags can be worn about the neck to keep you cool for hours. Plus they look very stylish if you ignore that as they melt they can drip on your clothes a little. But any of us used to dealing with baby drool can handle it. If the freezer makes them too cold, keep scarves in the refrigerator.

2.   Get some of those plastic spray bottles and load 'em up with cool water. These bottles come in different sizes from large to small enough to carry in your purse. When you feel the heat, spray your face of other body parts to cool off.

3.   When you can, keep your hair wet. Keeping your head cool helps to regulate your body temperature and feels wonderful. The same thing goes for hats! Soak your cotton hats in water and wear them about. If you think this makes you look too silly, think "How silly will I look when my symptoms bite me in the butt?"

4.   AIR CONDITIONING! Find it. Use it. Love it! Plan your events around areas that have air conditioning such as the movie theater, mall, or bookstore. Make sure to have your car's air conditioning checked before the days get hot so it doesn't conk out on you in the middle of summer. I found this out the hard way!

Here is another article from MS MINDS. It combines both serious ideas on trick-or-treating with the kids and some silly ideas for costumes.

Everyday is Not Halloween

It is coming again. The holiday, Halloween, when the ability to walk a mile in 10 minutes is prized highly among children. A time that invitations to dances and parties come blasting over the radio and through the mail. Halloween is not a sit down deal like Thanksgiving. It is not a "bask in the glow of the fireplace while the kids tear open boxes," holiday either. Moreover, unlike Easter, you are expected to go meandering about with your child as they hunt for their treats.

Many parents with MS or not, dread this holiday because of the physical intensity it can have. That and every paranoia we ever had about razor blades in apples comes back to haunt us. Here are some tips and ideas on how to make this Halloween Horribly Awesome!

Can't walk five blocks? Don't. Find a family your child can go trick or treating with that you trust. They can walk your child up and down the streets and you won't damper your child's night out by stopping because you're tired. Got older kids? Send the older ones out with the younger ones. You'll get an "Aww, Mom!" but bribe them with a percentage of candy or a night out.

If you do venture out, do not wear heavy costumes or masks. Masks not only block line of sight but also can be hot. The same with certain costumes. Sure, we know you wanted to be Barney for Halloween but all that purple fur gets very warm and we don't need you doing an impression of the fall of Rome.

When going out, make sure to map where you are going and

rest up the day before. Also, schedule time to be tired the next day if you take the chance of walking all over the neighborhood.

Find gatherings that are located in one place. Many community centers have Halloween Parties where children can get candy, do crafts, and run willy-nilly while you take it easy. Malls and other shopping areas often hand out candy and have activities for kids. They have many places to sit if you are not able to keep up.

If you use an electric wheelchair, why not dress it up? I know a man who attaches a dragons mask to the front of his and a tail to the back. Strap a mask on the front or stick a broomstick end coming out the back. Find a way to scoot along and be merry with your kids.

For those who simply cannot walk the blocks and have found alternative walkers for their kids, sit by the door and do the candy thing. However, instead of just being the lady who hands out candy, try to make your house a fun stop in the neighborhood. Make the front yard spooky. Have a treasure hunt for candy in your front yard. Rent a bouncy house and be the center of attention for your neighborhood Halloween night. But don't over do it physically. Get some help from your family and friends decorating before hand.

This leads me to my next suggestion. A neighborhood party. If you are close with your neighbors why not plan a street party? That way the kids can run about getting candy but it'll be in the same area.

Adult Parties (Not that kind!)

Yes, it has happened again. You've been invited to a Halloween party for grown ups with dancing. The last time you tried dancing was Uncle Louis' Polka Party and after you lost your footing and sprained your ankle, you've sworn to never put on your dancing shoes again. Not to mention how sore your legs were the next day. Day? Make that week.

So what do you do? Your husband wants to go out and you would rather sit by the door and give out candy. You have a few choices.

1. Wear a costume that you cannot possibly dance in. Whether it is dressing up as a box of Raisinets or replica of the Eiffel Tower, these costumes do not scream, "Come dance with me." When someone asks you, just say, "No, that's okay. I'll stand over here."

2. Only the slow songs. We all know how to shuffle in place, put it to good use. You get to hold on to someone for balance, and remember, it was his foot not yours! In addition, you get to shuffle back and forth and easily make it through the song. No one could say you didn't dance!

3. Run the bar. Alternatively, buffet table. Put yourself to use. Get behind the buffet table or punch bowl and dish out food and drinks. Whoever is throwing the party will be glad to have your help.

4. If you want to dance, go for it. In fact, give it your all and worry about the consequences tomorrow. For those of you still mobile, suck it up and be the woman your husband married. Laugh, joke, and who cares if you look a bit off balance or silly? You are having fun! Just remember my earlier advice about the next day and leave it open for resting.

Silly Ideas for MS costumes

The Myelin Mistress: Wrap yourself in cellophane from head to toe. Don't forget air-holes. This is another good way to avoid dancing or any other sort of movement. You are the nerve the cellophane is the nerve covering. This also works if you dress up as a hotdog. The bun is the myelin the dog is the nerve. But most people won't get it.

Crazy White Cell: If only they had a white M&Ms because the round costumes they put out for being M&Ms would be perfect for a white cell! Whether you dress completely in white or find a round form to put yourself in, make sure you get the foam for your mouth so you can get that rabid look. After all, you are after the myelin. Think Pacman.

The Brain: I don't know if I need to say more. Get a big brain hat to put on your head. Dress your child or husband as the white cell and have fun.

Hypodermic Needle: I have actually seen these costumes before (and no it wasn't in some freaky sci-fi dressing room). Simply use cloth pens to write your drug of choice "Betaseron, Copaxone, Rebif, Avonex" down the front and go out as your medicine.

The Nutty Neuro: Doctor's coat, stethoscope, and a grisly face made up with green and fangs. Add a bag full of empty pill jars filled with M&Ms. It's our worst nightmare of a nutty neurologist. Muhahahahaha!

Zombie: As discussed in a previous chapter, this is a way to show people exactly what MS fatigue does. Sallow face paint and shuffling. Heck, you may not even need to change your clothes. The MS Fatigue Zombie!

All right, just for those of you who may be thinking I am truly out of my head, these suggestions are merely to make you giggle not to be taken seriously. Although I just may go for the white cell costume. However I am also considering the Nutty Neuro for my get up this year. I know, morbid.

This is another article with advice for tackling the holidays. In the wintertime when the heat has passed, many of us still fall prey to flare-ups or relapse because of the stress brought on by the holidays. This first Christmas article is serious in its advice while, the one that follows entitled "What I'm Doing Next Year" is a bit sassier. Both were in MS MINDS, my newsletter that goes out in a completely erratic rhythm. (I am hoping to get it more regular, MS allowing!)

The MS of Christmas

Christmas with Multiple Sclerosis. No big deal right? We spend everyday with it, so why should the Christmas be any different? The holidays, just like summer time, come with certain pitfalls that can make it difficult for us to live with our MS.

Stress is the main cause of worsening symptoms around the holiday season. That and spiked eggnog overdose, but we'll discuss that another day. Once we grow from children to adults, Christmas can change from a thrilling holiday to a nail-biting, fast-paced, gift-wrapping, ham-roasting, tree-trimming, house-lighting, stress mess. This type of emotional and physical stress although weathered with ease by your average civilian, can be devastating to your average MSer.

Although it has not been scientifically proven that stress can worsen MS symptoms, many doctors warn their patients about its adverse effects. The aggravation of symptoms when a person is undergoing times of stress may come from a weakening in the person's system while the body tries to handle the added strain. I may not know why our symptoms intensify with stress but I do have some ideas on how to alleviate and avoid stress over the holidays.

1.   Say "NO." Too many of us are constantly taking on the projects and problems of those around us. I do not know exactly why this seems to be extra true with MSers, but I

believe that it must come from the fact that MSers are some of the most caring, loving people in the world. Watch yourself and look at your "to-do" list for this holiday. Have you taken on too much? Do you really need to bake 100 cookies and decorate each of them by hand? Do you really need to bake a fruitcake for Aunt Edna? Does that plastic Santa really have to be attached to the roof this year? No it doesn't. When you find yourself adding extra things to your list, stop and take a moment to decide whether or not it really needs to be done. Say no. I give you permission to say no, guilt free this holiday. This is a time for joy and loving, if someone gets grumpy with you about not doing something, just hit them upside the head with a fruitcake. It ought to knock some sense into them. Considering most people's fruit cakes, it could knock them unconscious as well.

2.   Take ONE shopping trip. Yes ONE. You heard me. I don't want to hear about the fact that you might forget something or how the stores you need to visit are in different locations all over town. First, if you haven't been buying most of your gifts over the Internet in your PJs while you relax with a cup of cocoa, you deserve to be looked at with that stern, disapproving mother look. I am squinting my eyes at you as I write this. Second, plan one trip. Okay maybe I will give you two trips, but try to do everything in one swoop, so that you can sit back and relax, knowing that your shopping is done. Write down the gifts you need to buy and the places you want to go and then plot them out so that you or your caretaker can drive in one circle. This way you are not zigzagging all over town using up gas and your energy. Once you have done this, you will feel less pressured and you will be more able to enjoy the approaching holiday.

3.   Simplify. Forget the lights on the roof. Let someone else play Indiana Jones on your roof tiles, while you relax in a lounge chair on the driveway and yell instructions. Ask your caretaker or friends to help with the decorating. Having MS does not

mean you should give up your holiday traditions, but it does mean that it may be time to swallow your pride, admit that you've never been anything like Martha Stewart, and ask for help.

4.   Spend more, work less.
        A.   Why not buy the cookies instead of making them? The people at the Christmas party will never know the difference. And who knows? There is the slim possibility that they have never liked your cooking and were only eating the stuff to be nice. Holidays really bring out our susceptibility to guilt.

        B.   If you feel the irresistible pull to send out Christmas cards, look into having them pre-printed to give your hands a rest.

        C. Shop online, and pay the extra shipping fees to avoid the crowded store and the physical onslaught of symptoms you will experience by being there. Walking up and down aisles in crowded stores, which are usually noisy and hot, can only make you worse. Heck, even non-MSers can get sick due to the crowds.

        D. If the grand family Christmas gathering, complete with aunts and uncles, is normally at your house, think about having it at some other family member's home. This will take a great deal of stress off you and give you more time to enjoy the holiday with those you love. Give someone else the joy of explaining to Aunt Edna why you didn't make the Christmas ham with her recipe and the thrill of cleaning up the mess after the Smith twins have experimented with how much toilet paper can go down in one flush. These sweet memorable occasions can be passed on to some other unsuspecting family member so that you can sit back and relax. Not to mention, you can chuckle softly to yourself when the Smith twins head upstairs with that mischievous look in their eyes.

5.   Spend less, work some. With this option you will be doing a bit more but spending less money. Try making your gifts. You can give the same gift of a wonderful batch of homemade cookies, soaps, or wreaths to everyone on your list, or you can make special gift baskets designed with each person in mind. Gift baskets are inexpensive, as they can be filled with lots of little things with a certain theme in mind. For example you can pick the person's favorite color and buy them items in only that shade or you can pick a certain hobby of theirs and work with that. Here are two examples:

A. Purple Basket. Many craft stores carry various styles of low priced baskets with which to start your gift. In addition, at the craft store you can pick up a few purple flowers and some purple tissue paper to line the basket. You can find some purple candles in various sizes and put them in the basket. Depending on the winters in your part of the country, you could add a purple scarf and mittens. A pair of warm, toasty socks would be a welcomed gift to anyone no matter the weather. Purple soaps, trinket boxes, body oils, hair accessories, candies, and live flowers are all items that can be added to your basket. This basket, depending on what you add to it can cost $15 to $30.

B. For the Friend who Loves Romance Novels get a white wicker basket, or one with a rose colored hue to it. Add one or two romance novels, a box of tissues with a nice design on it (for those scenes that make her weepy), a candle for reading chocolates to go with the sinful parts, and a bookmark with a saying that lets her know how much you care. You can even make one of your own with some pretty paper. I was able to put one these baskets together for only $20.

C. The tool basket. Buy some various tools and other parts you can't even name, and put them not in a wicker basket, but instead shove them into a tackle box or inexpensive plastic toolbox. This should satisfy the one question your husband or male friend always seems to be asking, "Where is my

1/2 inch wrench?"

These are just a few tips on how to curb your stress this Christmas. By following just a few simple rules and with a few new gift ideas under your belt, you should be well prepared. Remember, saying NO, condensing your shopping trips and economizing can make this Christmas less panic and more celebration of the joy of living and loving as it was meant to be

This was the second article written years following my first Christmas with MS. (Note the subtle differences. One is helpful and one is sarcastic.) However this being a rant and a blast from the past, I just had to re-print it for your reading pleasure.

Next Year I'll Remember: More Christmas Ideas

I made it through Christmas. I even went shopping on, *gasp,* Christmas Eve! Of course, if I'd had my old memory, I wouldn't have forgotten so many things and had to go back out on the 24th. But hey, such is life with MS. I survived the holiday parties, the hectic shopping trips, the horrible weather, and the relatives. Bets are still being placed on whether or not I make it through New Years.

However, there are a few points I'm going to remember for next year. This means I have to type them out or they'll be erased from my brain's filing system by next Christmas.

I will remember to consider shoe choices carefully before attending parties. Balance problems, wine, and clogs don't mix. This should have been an easy one, but silly me had to nearly break her neck before she noted the bad shoe choice. In my mind clogs didn't count as heels so I was in the clear. Add with my already wobbly balance, two glasses of wine, blend in a throw rug and you have a comedy routine waiting to happen. Thankfully, my sister was there to catch me. And I am still thanking the Powers That Be for the lack of anyone with a video camera at that moment.

I will remember that list making does not help if you forget the list. Next year I vow either to make a knit sweater with my shopping list crocheted on to it, or to staple the list to my butt. Hey, I poke myself with needles all the time, a little stapling shouldn't be much of a change, right? All helpful MS sites, including my own, talk about making lists and such. But honestly, with the added stress of the holidays, expect to forget the list. When you get to the store and have no list, you're left wandering the aisles with a blank look attempting to remember not only what was on the list, but also where you left it. So next year I will attempt the following procedure with my list:

A. Give the list to my husband. If he forgets it, I can barrage him with guilt and walk around with my halo on, because I wasn't the one who messed up.

B. Cover myself with sticky notes.

C. Put the list in my mouth. You know half hanging out, not all the way in your mouth. That way as I am running out the door, grabbing the mail, coats, and keys, I will not put the list down on the counter where I will end up leaving it.

I will remember to get everyone the same thing. Sure the kids may not find playing with socks all that fun, but you'll have everyone covered and there are many uses for socks. They can be cell phone covers, puppets, gloves, and well, socks. Dye the sock a festive color and shove candies in it. Wait! We already do that. Darn!

I will embrace gift bags. Lots and lots of gift bags. Okay, I was never any good with scissors anyhow, but now that I'm a bit unpredictable with sharp objects due to tremors, by the way, and not mood swings. Wrapping has become dangerous. Although my son thinks it's funny how Mommy talks to the wrapping paper and God while attempting this, so next year, its gift bags all the way. No scissors and you don't have to figure out how to get objects that are not square completely covered by practically unbendable paper.

I will remember fake trees. Yep. My husband was right. Once that puppy is loaded with ornaments no one ever noticed the difference. Oh, wait. Yes, they did. They noticed how I had no pine needles all over my floor, and I was not attempting what looks like a yoga pose to water the dang thing. My son likes building it. It's life size Legos to him. My husband didn't have to kill anything (He really does hate that), and I didn't find myself wishing for an SUV at the tree lot. Because I really do dislike those cars. Not in the country, where they are useful and people know how to drive them, but here in the city, where the drivers only use them for pushing small cars around and taking up two parking spaces. Okay I don't hate SUVs, just most of the drivers.

I will remember to reread my own articles on how to deal with Christmas!

Those are my thoughts of what I'm going to either keep doing or do differently next year. I'm sure I'll come up with a few more to lessen the stress and exhaustion of the holidays, like enjoy my family, and not be sucked in by commercials, but for now this list will do. Hopefully, I won't forget it.

Kids and MS: Ideas for telling them

A mother once asked me how I told my young son about my Multiple Sclerosis. "How do you explain that some days you are always in bed or sick?" She was very frustrated and upset. After Mommy had been sick for a week, her five-year-old son was getting worried and she didn't know how to describe what was going on. She needed help, but was not getting the answers she wished from her doctors. "They all tell me that he is on a need to know basis, and to only tell him what he needs to know. I can't even begin to think of how to explain the complex workings of MS and the brain. I'm not sure he even knows what a brain is!" When this email flashed across my screen I completely understood what she was going through.

In my first book, *Coffee in the Cereal*, I shared my first attempt at telling my eldest son, Stephan, about my MS. I also reminded everyone that I am not a doctor or a psychologist and I do not know what will happen to his psyche because of the way I explained my disease to him. If someday I am called to rescue him from a local hospital where they have him strapped up in a room yelling, "KILL ALL WHITE CELLS!" then I will admit defeat and shut my mouth. But until that happens, I will continue to give advice to mothers, who after finding my website for moms with MS (MS Moms), still send me frantic emails asking for advice.

In my opinion, friends are often exceedingly more helpful than doctors are when it comes to parenting. I recall how much help I received from my pediatrician when Stephan was a baby, "Yep. That's a boy all right!" and the good advice from my friends, "Put down the thermometer and step away from the Dr. Spock! Now go to the neighborhood park, sit back, and learn." Swimming pools, parks, grocery stores, these are the places to learn child rearing. That said, you may understand why I look to my friends for parenting ideas more often than the oh-so eloquent doctor. Of course I am not condoning that you never listen to, or visit, a doctor again. I wouldn't be so silly.

When it comes to telling our children about MS however, I think other parents with MS are one of the best places to look. Even if their advice is not from a clinical study or a 10-year college degree, it is from experience. On a message board you can get over 10 different answers on how to do something. Doctors can only give one. Besides they are interested in dealing with your MS. Their job title does not necessarily include how to deal with your family. If they do help, count yourself lucky.

As a friend, let me share the many different ways I have for telling my son about my MS. Before we start, I have to express that it took descriptions in many different ways and on different occasions before it really sunk in for my son. Even now, at the age of 9, we still have little refresher courses when Mommy goes down after being okay for awhile. Do not expect your child to instantly "get it" and not forget it.

These ideas are mainly for young children (ages 5 and up). Older children and teenagers are going to have a better grasp of the human body and will most likely be able to handle straight forward descriptions. The very young (ages 1-4) may not be able to understand the descriptions. It is always difficult to decide what to tell your child at any age, but especially when our children are younger. I ask parents to use their best judgment and knowledge of their own children when deciding what they wish to take and use from my ideas.

Ways to explain MS to your children:
Start with the basic information on how a regular body works.

The Brain

First, draw Mr. Stick Figure. Make a big circle for the head. Draw another circle or kidney bean shape inside the head. This is Mr. Stick's brain. Circle the brain and talk about how it is in the head and how it controls everything our body does. For older kids the words "command center" come to mind. Next, draw lines from the brain to different parts of the body, i.e., the hands, feet, legs. Explain that through these lines, or nerves, Mr. Stick's brain sends messages, or orders, to the parts of the body.

How do the nerves work?

During one of Mommy's MS lectures, I attempted to use the phone to explain how nerves transmit messages. My son, Stephan, didn't get it. So we moved on to his remote control car. I had him hold the controller and told him it was the brain. Then we attached some strings from his remote to the car itself to act as nerves. Some remote control cars have a wire attached to them from the car to the controller. This is a great example of a nerve, without taping strings to the car. When my son moved the joystick one way or another, we talked about those messages went down the string to the car to tell it what to do. The strings were the nerves and the remote the brain. He is a visual learner. If your child is able to grasp the concept that we can't see the nerves taking the messages, you can remove the strings on the car. Now comes the part where you explain how MS affects your body, when the message doesn't go through.

Damaged nerves

Next, I began to fray and cut some of the strings attached to the car. If you are using the car with a wire already attached, I don't suggest fraying the wire unless you want to risk ruining your car or being zapped. While my son was in the bathroom, I took out one of the batteries to better explain my idea. When he came back, he tried to get the "brain" to tell the "body" what to do. The car did not move. I explained that this is what happens when those nerves from the brain to the body are damaged, as they can be in Multiple Sclerosis.

Another way to explain how the messages do not get through is to take a long wrapping paper tube and talk through it to your child. Then if you begin to cut the tube or break it, the sound changes and the message is not as clear. If he is interested in walkie-talkies, try changing the frequencies and noticing on which channel the message gets through the best, then switching channels and showing how the sound breaks up. You can do this with TV channels as well.

Finally, explain that when those messages don't get through, it causes your body to do funny things and makes you sick. Though it is a bit farfetched, you can tell your child that the "be awake" message is not getting through today. The same with the "move legs" message.

How were the nerves damaged?
One way to explain what happens to the nerves and the myelin, as well as describe what they are, is to get out an Oreo cookie. Give most children an Oreo and the first thing they do is twist off the top of the cookie, heading for that creamy center. Just like little raging white cells, heading for the creamy center under the myelin of your nerves. If your child does this, it is a good time to pause and explain to them that your nerves are covered by coats, like the cover of the Oreo and that the inside of your nerves, are like the creamy filling. Next, you can point out that your child did exactly what your MS causes the "bad guys" to do. They rip off the nerve coat to get to the center. They want to rip off that crunchy coating and get to the good stuff at the center. Okay, so my son Stephan looked simultaneously guilty and horrified, but he got the point, momentarily. Then he was sidetracked and wanted to know if our nerves looked like Oreos and how they tasted. Some children are more literal than others are.

Alternatively, you can use the Oreo like this: The myelin is the cookie outside and the nerves are the mushy white inside. If you chip at the cookie cover, the white (nerve) becomes exposed. Take the top off and drop the cookie on the ground. Dirt gets all over the white filling and that shows how the nerve is not protected. Talk about how a dirty nerve might be bad at sending correct messages.

Another way to explain unprotected nerves is with one of those ice cream cones with a chocolate shell. You can poke at the chocolate gently with a toothpick and the ice cream is still okay, but if you remove large chunks of the covering or all of it, then the ice cream can melt and fall out. It is now damaged. These ideas may help explain how the myelin protects the nerves.

Of course with the ice cream experiment when the ice cream began dripping out of the chocolate holes, Stephan wanted to know why he never saw my nerves hanging out of my body. I explained that our skin keeps our nerves in and he asked why when I got a cut, a nerve didn't hang out. When I said that the nerves were further under the skin and not close to the surface he bluntly asked how then, could he "get on my nerves?" This was yet another time for Mommy to almost expire from choking on coffee, while trying not laugh.

What exactly is damaging the nerves (or creamy coating)? Trying to explain white cells and an immune system gone awry is rather difficult. Kids have a hard enough time grasping the brain sending messages down broken nerve lines, let alone trying to understand the complexity of our immune system and our cells. Trust me you don't want to get into a discussion about the difference between prison cells and blood cells and then an argument about why both are spelled the same way.

With Stephan at age 9, I am just beginning to get into an explanation of our immune system and how it works. Mr. Literal and I are still having heated discussions about cells are, why they are in our bodies.

"Mommy, then how come you have a cell phone?" The ensuing cell phone discussion had him freaked out, because he suddenly wondered if our mobile phones (Lord, why hadn't I used the word mobile in the first place?) were powered by blood.

So, skip the immune system explanation and just pit the good guys against the bad guys. If your child wants to know who the good guys and bad guys are you can just say they are parts in your body. Pray your child does not need to know what parts and their specific names. I think most children however, will accept general answers.

Think of a TV show or movie that your child loves, one that has clear set of good guys and bad guys. For my son at age six it was Pokemon. I used Ash, Misty, and Brock against Team Rocket and Meowth from the show. I tried to explain MS by pitting the good guys (my medicine) against the bad guys (the raging white cells.) The bad guys want to destroy the nerve coatings and the good guys must stop them. Since explaining the white cells as "misguided," which is closer to the truth, might prove too confusing for a child, just be absolute, and make them bad guys. It's a simple concept that children can grasp and process quickly. In my case I never had to explain cells to my son at all, I just told him there was a battle going on in my body and he accepted it. I wish adults were as easy to get along with.

Always assure your child that the bad guys are not winning. Remind your child that like in most of their favorite movies, bad guys never win. Unless they're running for some governmental office.

If you do take some form of medicine for your MS, explain that the medicine is the good guys. When my son accidentally burst in while I was giving myself a shot, I calmly told him, "This is the way I shoot the good guys into my body so they can go attack the bad guys." Being a typical boy, now he wants to watch every time I take my shot so he can cheer on the good guys. Mommy is having a hard time deciding whether it is appropriate for him or not. Then again what could be more frightening then Teletubbies? For young children, the bad guys don't have to be killed or attacked, just put in time-out for eternity.

The basics I recommend remembering:
1. There is a battle going on in your body. On the other hand, some cells are just being brats by not doing what they have been told to do.

2. Nerves tell your body what to do and are protected by coats. When he goes out during winter with a jacket on, he is protected from the cold the same way the myelin protects the nerves from damage.

3. When the coat is damaged or removed, the nerve is exposed and the messages don't get through correctly. When he runs off without a jacket in rainy weather, he is unprotected and gets wet and cold, just as unprotected nerves are damaged.

4. You are not going to die. Your child may need to hear this many times.

5. The medicine you take, or if you don't take any explain you have good cells that are battling the confused cells, stops the bad guys. Alternatively, it gets rid of the bad guys who are trying to take off the nerve coats.

6. There will be days when the bad guys seem to be winning. On those days Mommy or Daddy will not be feeling good. The best thing for your child to do is help you rest. Many children love to help and will feel more in control when they can be

involved instead of banned from the room.

These ideas are just that: IDEAS. As I said before, I am not a professional, just a mom who has been explaining MS to her eldest for 4 years now. I didn't have a choice about when to tell him. Stephan overheard people talking about my MS and also heard them mention death. He became very afraid and Mommy had to do some quick thinking to ease his fears. Multiple Sclerosis can be difficult for us to understand let alone our children. Depending on the extent of your condition, you may not need to offer an explanation until your children are much older.

For those MSers who experience debilitating symptoms and long periods of relapse, you may have no choice but to find some way of explaining what is happening. Take some time to think about your child and how they process information. Think about what games or characters they like. This can help you to come up with ideas on how to go about explaining MS and your symptoms. For extra ideas check out the various MS websites and message boards. Here you can read articles and ask other parents how they did the telling.

This article was previously published on my MS MOMS website and in my MS MINDS newsletter. It approaches the subject of how to simplify things at home so that you can still feel like supermom. (Even though we all know that even those without the challenge of MS are not supermom! And simply being there for your kids and having fun with them is much more important than whether the laundry is finished or dinner is a masterpiece!) Some of my readers may already know this article but it needs publishing for those who have not seen it and need some advice on how to tackle the house. It also illustrates some of the topics we discuss at MS MOMS.

The Mother Load

So you have MS?
So what. Gimme my breakfast.
Where's my clean shirt? Where are my shoes?
Why is the house a mess? Bobby's hitting me!
He did it first! MOM!!!!!

Most mothers can identify with this. For many of us, this is a daily occurrence. The children still need raising and our husbands still can't find the car keys.

When we were first diagnosed with MS, they told us to "listen to our bodies" and to "rest when we needed it." Somewhere in the back of our minds, we remember the same advice when we held our first born in the hospital. There was no time for the advice then, and we sure as heck don't have it now. How can you listen to your body, when you can't even hear yourself speak over the clamor of family?

Many of us work at home these days. There are even some still out there working AND raising a family. (To those women, I bow my head in reverence. You're doing more than I can.) The concept of an MS mom resting in her bed when she needs to, while the kids clean the house and her husband cooks dinner after a long day at work, is a complete fallacy. (If you have a husband and kids like this, please give me your address. I know a couple scientists and not a few women that would like to examine and clone them.)

For most of us, the world didn't stop when we got MS. The house didn't begin to clean itself. The kids didn't somehow become little adults that walked about saying "Gee Mom, we have been selfish children. Since you need rest, we'll cook dinner and do the laundry." (Once again: if you have these kids, I have a laboratory that wants them.) The kids are still kids, the house is still a mess, and (in the case of those of us who had to give up working) our mate is the breadwinner. So who's left to take care of everyone? You.

MS moms don't get to stop. I am sure you have tried it. You laid on your bed closed your eyes and the laundry buzzer went off. You thought, "it'll keep," and closed your eyes again. Then came the phone call; you let the machine get it. As you began to relax, you heard the familiar stomping feet of your child searching you out. Lying on your bed, you keep your eyes closed tight and think, "Please let them not find me." The door creaks open. The voice that you love so much reaches your ears with some desperate plea for help, that only you can fix. Toys, siblings, homework, food, you pick. You sigh deeply and get back up. Wow! You listened to your body, and got 45 seconds of rest!

Since a mother doesn't get to stop being a mother when she gets MS, you need all the help you can get! The following tips have worked for me in tackling daily work and finding time to rest.

PUT WHEELS ON IT
If you have problems with weakness and fatigue (who doesn't?), lifting heavy laundry baskets, and lugging cleaning supplies about can wreak havoc on your body. Get a wagon. A simple

kid's wagon from the local toy store will do. If you have a toddler or preschooler at home, they may enjoy pulling the wagon about themselves. Use the wagon to hold anything you don't want to carry. The wagon works wonders for moving groceries from the car to the house. Love gardening? The wagon, if rugged enough, can easily move from housework to yard work.

I got rid of my son's toy box and bought simple wooden crates that came equipped with wheels. Now he can wheel the crate to wherever he's left his toys, and clean them up himself. If he doesn't, the darn thing has wheels and I can move it.

SIMPLIFY
Yes, you've heard this, but some of these ideas have really worked for me. Buy paper plates and cups! So your table doesn't look like Martha Stewart's and your friend's raise their eyebrows. If you don't have energy for the dishes, your mate is just home from work, and the kids have done their share, why not use paper? Do you want to do the dishes? You can eat your dinner and then just chuck the stuff into the trash. Since my husband has to work out of town on many weekends, this has helped me keep those dishes from piling up.

Make simple meals. You know there are going to be days when you don't have the energy to cook dinner. (For me, just about every single night!) Many grocery stores have meals that are already prepared. Just reheat and eat! Some of these include stir-fry meals that you can just plop in a pan and heat. Why not use a slow cooker? In the morning, when you have the most energy, you can toss the ingredients in and it will be ready by dinnertime.

Use throw rugs and runners. I hate mopping. It's the worst. Putting a runner carpet down in the area of the kitchen that gets the most traffic can help. In our house, the back door opens into the kitchen and there is always a track of footprints from that door across the floor. To solve the problem, we put a simple throw rug down, so instead of mopping, I can just clean the little rug. I hang it over the fence and blast it with a hose. A little rug in front of the sinks has helped immensely as well.

Nowadays you can get a Swiffer or some other electronic mop and these are great for a quick wipe down of the kitchen floor or halls without lugging a bucket and mop. If you use a mop & bucket see the above and get one with WHEELS!

CONSOLIDATE
Pick when you have the most energy in the day and set that time aside to get as much done as possible. Nobody said you have to finish it all, but you can easily get the dishwasher going, turn the washer on, and maybe vacuum one room, before you need a rest period. Then, after resting, you may be able to switch loads, and feel up to tackling another room. (The kids can empty the dishwasher. But if you used the paper plates, you didn't have dishes in the first place!)

For appointments and errands, try to make a big circle. Instead of driving from one end of town to the other and back again, pick one time of day to get it all done, and make a little map so that you drive efficiently. It took awhile for my husband and me to accomplish this, but now I schedule as many appointments as I can on one day, so that we aren't driving to an appointment every single day of the week. Since the store is near our son's preschool, we schedule any shopping while going to or from picking him up.

Try not to plan major activities too close to your appointment day. MS is like having a battery that needs recharging. Take a light day before your appointment day so that your battery is charged up for the day of running around. If you have any big event ahead of you, take a light day before it and be aware that the day after the event will likely be a down day. I learned at the State Fair one summer that not watching the weather channel and not taking a slow day before could be devastating. By the way, check your medicine. Besides already being sensitive to heat, I made the mistake of not noticing that my medicine made me MORE sensitive to heat and sun. I had a horrible time and could have wound up in the hospital. (Also, do not assume the brakes on all rental wheelchairs work!)

REMINDERS

Many of us have lost our time sense, or have the wonderful knack for forgetting nowadays. Make the egg timer your friend. Having little timers all over the house has helped me remember things like: "Oh, yeah! I have the oven on." After having a few too many cooking fires, my husband insisted I either use a timer or quit cooking. If you get a timer that can go for long amounts of time, you can set it to go off before you need to leave for an appointment or to pick up your kids.

Use message services. Companies will call you to remind you of things such as that appointment you're forgetting right now. Some of them even do wake up calls. Of course, they charge a fee for this service. But it can be invaluable.

Tack up the sticky notes. If you can find the type that doesn't fall off, sticky notes can be placed around the house to remind you of necessary chores. Pick different colors to represent different things, if you think you can remember what the color means.

REST

First things first. Unplug the phone! Don't listen to the machine either! For a small monthly fee, I have voice mail, so that when I unplug everything, I can still get messages. Speaking of phones, here in California the phone company offers a cordless phone for free if you don't already have one. It comes with a hook so you can wear it, and it saves you having to walk all over the house to answer it.

Anyway what was the next helpful hint? Oh yes, REST! Every

single bit of rest time helps. I know you are thinking this sounds as helpful as the old adage "sleep when the baby sleeps." Right! When the kids are napping or at school, we don't rest, admit it. We want to finish the housework, laundry, and get in a good, long hot shower! But try to conk out when you can. If you find yourself in the middle of the creating best casserole ever known to man and the fatigue hits, just stop it, drop it, and roll into bed! Unless you have it in the oven and then you use the timer I told you to buy. You can always finish it later.

Make sure the laundry buzzer isn't going to go off when you are resting, and put a note on your front door so people don't come calling. Make sure that there are no cats in your room, because they always want to cuddle just as you're about to doze off, and send the barking dog outside. Get an emergency pager that only the school or you husband can dial. Make sure that if you're interrupted, it's for a really good reason.

Plan your rest time. Don't try to rest when you know everyone will be searching you out. If you have a young child, rest when they take their naps. I know you are scoffing right now, but it can work. In fact I find more often than not with my newborn that when he passes out, I do to. With older children, when they first get home from school, they are usually interested in snacks and some playtime before homework. Have the snacks ready and then go lay down while they play. If you know your friends and neighbors well enough, you can even work out a time when they won't be knocking or mowing, so that you can relax.

Use "ooooo" machines. You know those things that make those un-natural nature sounds. Since I choose to rest when my husband is home to help with our sons, I bought a little sound machine that makes ocean sounds or even cricket chirps. Don't use this setting, trust me. The sound blocks the noise coming from the rest of the house and helps me relax. After I found that crickets and kids crying do not mix, I turned on my air-purifier. You know the ones loud enough to drown out jets? They can be perfect for making a white noise that blocks out everything. Add some ear plugs, a sleep mask, and you have complete sensory depravation to help you drift. (Of course many of us have to keep our ears open for our children's near-death experiences.)

DO IT IN BED OR ON THE COUCH! (No, this isn't THAT chapter.)

If it just seems that you're not going to get the chance to rest, become queen bee and do as much as you can while reclining in the hive. I read books to my son or let him watch TV in my room, while I lay back. Older children might enjoy doing their homework in the room with you while you lay back. If you have work you need to do, bill paying or anything else, do it in bed! Some of the lap desks are great for sitting in bed and having a hard surface to work on. Some of them even have slots on the side to hold materials. All of this can also be done from a couch as well.

Play Nintendo, cards, or board games. It's quality time with your children and doesn't require any serious physical exertion. Besides, you might enjoy it, and it helps exercise your hand to eye coordination. Or at least you can say that when your husband asks why you are playing the Pokemon Puzzle game when your son is at school.

None of us are going to be able to spend every day listening to our bodies and resting when we need to. Most of us are not rich, and do not have a maids or nannies. Take as much time as you can, and try a few of these tips. Every bit of help makes your load a bit lighter.

If you find your food burned, your laundry pink, and your refrigerator is ringing while your son runs about in mismatched socks, you might be trying too hard. If we try too hard to be super woman, it's usually a good bet that we're doing too much and chaos is going to break out. This is a big clue to choose what is important and what is not. I'd say a happy, healthy Mom is the most important thing for our families and ourselves. Not a frazzled, half-dead woman in pink socks. Wouldn't you?

A Woman's Touch: MS and Femininity

When was the last time you were proud of your body? Or the last time you felt sexy? If it was just recently, then I applaud you. Most of us with MS however may be shaking our heads and laughing sarcastically at this, thinking "Ya, was that a year ago or two years ago?"

MS can ravage a woman's sense of identity. Women MSers battling with fatigue, loss of sensation, and mobility problems, often find themselves loosing their sense of femininity. Weight gain caused by lack of mobility and fatigue can make this situation even worse.

A lot of us have the idea that people with disabilities are not attractive. Walking with a cane or being in a wheelchair can not only wreak havoc on your pride, but on your sense of feminine grace as well. Being sucked under by fatigue and loss of sensation, can make you feel less than sexy. Add bladder problems and spasticity on top of that and you're likely to feel horribly unattractive.

As I was watching TV and glancing through magazines, the idea of disability being unattractive was confirmed by the lack of disabled women represented in the media. When is the last time you saw a model in a wheelchair? Or a movie where the leading lady had speech problems and was numb on her left side? Currently, we have the popular TV drama West Wing where the president has MS, but the president is a man.

Having MS does not mean you have to lose yourself, girl. There is a beautiful, wild woman in there who is dying to get out. Here are a few helpful tips and reminders for reviving your self-esteem and sense of femininity.

1. Get rid of the media. If the magazines make you upset and remind you of all those things you can't do, THROW THEM AWAY! If the TV shows you watch are bringing you down, quit watching them. There is no sense in dragging yourself through the mud every time you see a Victoria's Secret ad. And Baywatch isn't good for anyone's self image in my opinion.

2. Remember that beauty is in the eye of the beholder. If you see yourself as ugly, then you will feel ugly. Embrace the beauty that is inside you. Notice what beautiful eyes you have or how graceful your hands are. Focus on your pluses, instead of your minuses.

3. Buy "lovies." Lovies are items that make you feel spoiled and feminine. For me it is this wonderful peppermint scented soap and a soft chenille blanket in deep blue. I soak in the lukewarm tub with my soap and then wrap myself in the blanket while I eat chocolates and read trashy romance novels. This small amount of pampering helps me get back in touch with myself. Pamper yourself. Lovies can be anything from perfume, clothing, chick-flicks, wonderful massages, or dinners at great restaurants.

4. Read books that make YOU feel magnificent. You do not need to spend everyday reading articles and books about your MS. Grab something like *Succulent Wild Woman* by Sark or her fantastic book *How to Change Your Life Without Getting Out of Bed.* It's a playful book about guilt free napping, which is something I personally have a hard time doing. Try a *Chicken Soup* series book, even! Find a book that reminds you about what a special person you are. Use it to stop wracking yourself with guilt and pain. Other good books are *Gift from the Sea* by Anne Morrow Lindbergh and *SoulWork* by

Bettyclare Moffatt. For new mothers, I suggest *The Girlfriend's Guide to Surviving the First Year of Motherhood* by Vicki Iovine. Alternatively, there is *Operating Instructions* by Anne Lamott. (Warning this book is not sugar-coated and shows real and sometimes negative emotion about raising your first child. I find it relaxing because of the truth it is not afraid to exhibit.)

5. Give yourself a spa night. Set some candles around your tub. Fill it up with bubbles, play some soothing music, grab your book, and slip in. If lukewarm baths are not your thing because hot water can make your symptoms flare, try a cozy relaxation in your room. Surround yourself with food you love, dress in an outfit that makes you feel sexy and just enjoy the time to celebrate being a woman.

6. Enlist your mate. Oftentimes MS puts a deep strain on relationships. Most likely your mate would love to glimpse the happy carefree woman you once were and would do almost anything to see her again. Take a country drive together. Go to an ice cream parlor or walk barefoot in your backyard at night (Okay maybe not if you have a dog.) Meet your mate for a rendezvous at a hotel or a meal at a romantic restaurant. Put on that silly lingerie thing with only one strap. You know, the one hiding in the back of your underwear drawer? You might feel silly. You might think you have changed too much, but you are still the woman he fell in love with, no matter if you can do acrobatics five times a night or not. Sometimes all he needs is to know you are willing to try.

These are just a few ideas to help regain a bit of your feminine self and to help you feel beautiful again. It may take time. Many of us have been dealing with MS for years and have started to feel asexual, but it can come back.

Just remember, MS may have changed your life, and your body, but it can never touch your soul.

Books:

Sark, 1997 *Succulent Wild Woman*
New York: Fireside
Sark, 1999 *Change Your Life Without Getting Out of Bed: The Ultimate Nap*Book.
New York: Fireside
Canfield, Jack 1997 *Chicken Soup for the Mother's Soul*
Florida: HCI
Canfield, Jack 1996 *Chicken Soup for the Woman's Soul*
Florida: HCI
Lindbergh, Anne Morrow 1991 *Gift from the Sea*
New York: Pantheon
Moffatt, Bettyclare 1994 *Soulwork: Clearing the Mind, Opening the Heart, and Replenishing the Spirit.*
California: Wildcat Canyon Press
Iovine, Vicki 1997 *The Girlfriend's Guide to Surviving the First Year of Motherhood.*
New York: Perigee Books
Lamott, Anne 1994 *Operating Instructions: A Journal of My Son's First Year*
New York: Ballantine Books

Dear Friend,

Symptom Free...
It is an extreme and unfair world. On one hand, there are people who find their life after a diagnosis of multiple sclerosis turned inside out and who spend day after day trying to regain some semblance of their previous existence. On the other, there are those who seem to have a way to live their lives, unaffected and symptom free. It's as if they've decided to live life on their own terms and have made their MS respond to them.

You may know some of these people. And my guess is... you'd like to be just like them. Now you can! For a limited time I am going to share with you the secrets of living a life of peaceful coexistence with MS! This knowledge was before only given to the highest ranking in the MS world. You know, those loaded with money. But now, you too, can experience the secrets of Living With It.

Live beyond a cure…
In this book you are not going to find the secrets to a life-long cure or a few vague Zen-like phrases to help you on your way. Instead, you are going to hear about life experiences and how I faced them with Multiple Sclerosis! You will be able to walk away from this book having learned how to face everyday situations with your MS, and a bit about how to deal with them.

Take a look…
Have you ever wondered how to help your co-workers recognize your fatigue? Just follow my instructions on how to paint your face like the walking dead and they'll understand in no time!

Have you ever been faced with the embarrassment of running into your own furniture? Don't waste any more time feeling like a klutz! In this book you will learn how to blame a family member by shouting "Who the heck moved the coffee table!" You see? Now, no one can say you're simply physically challenged! (This also works for any flailing outside the home. Simply shout "did you see that?" and quickly move yourself and whoever is walking with you quickly away before they can discover there was nothing there!) Don't you love it? Say you love it!

Multiple Sclerosis is a life long disease. Don't you think it's time you took charge of your life and got out of bed? Isn't it time to learn how to face those nasty government workers and come out smiling? I won't tell you how to get your disability payments, but I will tell you how to use your inner strength to smile in the face of adversity instead of using your cane as a weapon. It's all here in this book! And if you act now you'll get the free picture of the author you see here! So what are you waiting for? Purchase this book today and start living!

In the five years that I have lived with MS, I have discovered the single most important piece of information a person will need to know in order to find peace and I'm going to reveal it to you right now. Because the rest of this book has nothing to do with this tongue-in-cheek intro:

How do you handle your life with MS?

Just like you handled it last month, only completely different.